Nursing Adults with Respiratory Disorders

Nursing Adults with Respiratory Disorders

Edited by

Jane E. Scullion

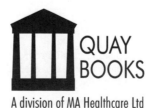

QUAY
BOOKS

A division of MA Healthcare Ltd

Quay Books Division, MA Healthcare Ltd, St Jude's Church, Dulwich Road, London
SE24 0PB

British Library Cataloguing-in-Publication Data
A catalogue record is available for this book

© MA Healthcare Limited 2007

ISBN-10: 1 85642 311 5
ISBN-13: 978 1 85642 311 3

Printed by Athenaeum Press Ltd, Dukesway, Team Valley, Gateshead, SE11 0PZ

Contents

Contents

Preface

There is clearly a considerable burden on health care, the economy, and individual patients and their carers as a result of respiratory diseases. In the United Kingdom, one in five deaths occurs as the result of respiratory disease, with more deaths occurring from this group of disease than from coronary heart disease or non-respiratory cancers. The UK death rate from respiratory disease is one of the highest in Europe (estimated to be around twice the European Union average) and it appears that this is a burden which is increasing, in contrast with coronary heart disease, where the relative burden is falling. However, it is the morbidity and the health costs of respiratory disease that have enormous consequences for individuals and the health services. It is estimated that around one in eight admissions to the acute sector is a consequence of respiratory disease, and there are also many consultations and house calls in primary care.

This book looks at the more common respiratory diseases that are seen, both in the hospital sector and in primary care. It is written by specialists involved directly in patient care. It is not an exhaustive manual, given the breadth and range of respiratory disorders with which patients present, but it does detail the more common presenting problems and their care, management and treatment. Each chapter is useful as a standalone text and contains a full list of references. What is apparent is that respiratory patients present in all specialties and that all health care professionals will look after patients with respiratory conditions, either as an acute event or as the consequence of chronic disease. It is hoped that this will be a useful reference book for students, nurses and other health care professionals with an interest in respiratory disease and its care, management and treatment.

Jane E. Scullion
April 2007

Contributors

Sue Burton
Respiratory Nurse Specialist
From a previous background working with patients requiring nasal ventilation, Sue Burton joined the early discharge scheme in the hospital and more recently developed and leads the Respiratory Early Discharge Scheme (REDS) for patients with COPD.

Jan Chantrell
Asthma/Allergy Nurse Specialist
Jan is an Asthma Nurse Specialist at the Glenfield Hospital, heading a team of nurses and with a personal interest in allergy. Her post at the hospital is part-time, complemented by her role as Head of Allergy at Education for Health.

Alison Conway
Respiratory Nurse Practitioner
Alison Conway, RN, BSc (Hons), has worked in the field of respiratory medicine for the past 15 years and has a wealth of experience in this area. She was a regional trainer for the National Respiratory Training Centre for ten years and has published extensively, both nationally and internationally. She was a scientific advisor to the World Health Organization in their publication *Adherence to Long-Term Therapies* on the basis of her previous work in this area. She currently woks as a nurse practitioner on the Clinical Decisions Unit at Glenfield Hospital and jointly runs a nurse-led haemoptysis clinic, where patients may be discharged at first contact.

Liz Darlison
Respiratory Nurse Consultant
As a Nurse Consultant in Mesothelioma, Liz has a wealth of experience of nursing as a practice development nurse, and more recently in patient care

moving from a role as lung cancer nurse specialist to her present position. She has developed the UK Mesothelioma Centre based at Glenfield Hospital, which has developed as a specialist centre for both patients and other health care professionals.

Berni Donaghy
Cystic Fibrosis Nurse Specialist
Berni developed the role of Cystic Fibrosis Nurse Specialist within the respiratory unit and works as a fundamental member of the multidisciplinary team involved in the care, management and treatment of patients with cystic fibrosis.

Karen Duncan
Respiratory Nurse Practitioner
Karen Duncan is married with one son and is currently expecting her second child. She has worked within the cardio-respiratory speciality for 20 years. After having been a ward manager in cardiology she moved back to respiratory care and worked as a practice development nurse. Karen was one of the first Modern Matrons in Leicester and went on to undertake the role of Assistant Head of Nursing. It was during this time that she successfully gained her MSc in Advanced Nursing Care at Nottingham University. Recently Karen decided to focus her career within a more dedicated clinical role and is currently a Respiratory Nurse Practitioner in a busy Clinical Decisions Unit. She has a wide range of clinical skills and expertise and is also enjoying the challenge of studying for a second MSc in Clinical Sciences at Leicester University.

Jo Hargrave
Education and practice development nurse, Thoracics, Respiratory and HDU
Jo has extensive experience as an Education & Practice development nurse working in thoracics, respiratory medicine and the HDU areas in these specialities and developing the skills of the nursing staff.

Theresa Harvey
BSc, PGDip Phys, MCSP
Theresa is currently working on the Clinical Decisions Unit at Glenfield Hospital as an extended scope respiratory physiotherapist involved in the immediate assessment of acute patients.

Sarah Lea
Respiratory Nurse Practitioner
Sarah Lea works as a respiratory nurse specialist with chronic obstructive pulmonary disease patients. Based at Glenfield hospital and working in Leicester city, proving long term support to patients in the community. Sarah spent 17 years in primary care first as a district nurse then practice nursing with a special interest in respiratory care. A nurse prescriber since 2000 firstly with the D/N formulary, then in the first group in the midlands to undertake the independent and supplementary prescribing course in 2003.

Mike Morgan
Consultant Respiratory Physician
Mike is the clinical director for the respiratory unit at Glenfield Hospital and is responsible for the initiation and success of the many specialist posts within the department. He is a world renowned expert in pulmonary rehabilitation and has worked extensively with the British Lung Foundation and Breathe Easy patient groups. Currently he is part of the steering group for the COPD NSF development, and co-chairs the subgroups for end of life, stable disease and pulmonary rehabilitation.

Karen Payne
Bronchiectasis Nurse Specialist
From a background as a sister within the unit, Karen developed the role of Bronchiectasis Nurse Specialist and supports patients requiring intravenous therapies to undertake this in their own homes to enable them to continue with their lives outside of the hospital environment.

Ivy Rushby
Respiratory Nurse Specialist
Ivy Rushby (RN, RM) has been in practice for many years, at least twenty of them in respiratory nursing. At present she works as Respiratory Nurse Specialist as the founding member of an outreach specialist respiratory intervention team providing long-term support and admission prevention for patients with COPD.

Jane E. Scullion
Respiratory Nurse Consultant
Jane Scullion is a Respiratory Nurse Consultant working across the interface of primary and secondary care, primarily with patients with complex needs

resulting from their lung disease and also in the development of respiratory services. She currently sits as a member of the IMPRESS group, a collaboration between the GPIAG and the BTS looking at the future of service provision in light of changes in commissioning of services, and is on subgroups of the NSF for COPD looking at patient-focused outcomes, stable disease and end of life. In addition she has an honorary post at the Aberdeen department of General Practice and Primary Care and is both a trustee and facilitator for Respiratory Education UK.

Helen Thuraisingam
TB Nurse Specialist
Helen Thuraisingam trained at the North Middlesex Hospital in London in the early 1980s and moved to Leicester in 1987. She worked as a practice nurse with a special interest in asthma in primary care from 1995 and obtained a degree in Community Health Nursing in 1998. Between April 1998 and January 2002 Helen was employed as a Clinical Nurse Specialist in Communicable Disease Control and Public Health at Leicestershire Health Authority. During that time Helen was responsible for coordinating a team of nurses and health visitors managing a large outbreak of TB in a Leicester school.
Since 2002, she has been employed by Eastern Leicester Primary Care Trust, leading the Specialist TB Nursing Service. Helen is currently completing an MSc in Advanced Nursing Practice at the University of Nottingham.

D. D. Vara
Head of Cardiorespiratory Physiology
D. D. heads both the respiratory and cardiology physiological measurements departments at Glenfield Hospital and has a wealth of knowledge on all aspects of physiological measurements in these areas. His department supports the many varied respiratory services in the hospital.

Jo Williams
Pulmonary Rehabilitation Coordinator
Jo is the Senior Pulmonary Rehabilitation Specialist at Glenfield Hospital and has presented and published both nationally and internationally on the subject of pulmonary rehabilitation.

CHAPTER 1

Anatomy and physiology of the respiratory system

Karen Duncan

An understanding of the anatomy and physiology of the respiratory system is essential for understanding many of the disease processes that comise respiratory disorders.

The purpose of the respiratory system is the carriage of oxygen throughout the body and the transport of carbon dioxide so that it can be eliminated. It also helps to regulate the pH of the body.

The structure of the respiratory system can be split into two: the conduction zone and the respiratory zone (Figure 1.1).

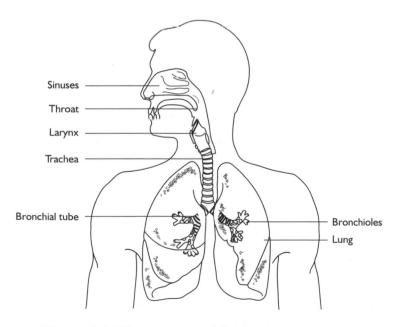

Figure 1.1 The structure of the respiratory system.

Conduction zone

These are the parts of the respiratory system which are filled with air (the anatomical dead space) but are not involved in gaseous exchange. During normal inspiration/expiration at rest (tidal volume) the volume of air moved is 500 ml. Of this, 150 ml fills the anatomical dead space, leaving 350 ml available for ventilation.

Respiration begins in the nose. Air enters the system via the nares (nostrils). The nose has a rich supply of blood vessels and is lined with ciliated columnar epithelium, which contains goblet cells that secrete mucus. The cilia move in a wave-like motion to waft dust and bacteria towards the throat, where they are then swallowed and nullified by the acid in the stomach or expectorated. This process is described as the mucociliary escalator. The conchae or turbinates form the walls of the nasal cavity as well as the convoluted channels called meatus. These serve to increase the surface area, allowing for the inspired air to be warmed, moistened and filtered effectively. Ducts called paranasal sinuses open into the internal part of the nose. They help with the vibration of sound when speaking and reduce the overall weight of the skull.

Pharynx (throat)

This is a passage connecting the nasal cavity with the larynx and the mouth with the oesophagus, allowing air and food to pass. Anatomically the pharynx can be divided into three sections: nasopharynx, oropharynx and laryngopharynx.

Larynx (voice box)

The vocal cords are situated here and are essential for producing sound. The larynx is a short tube located at the base of the hyoid bone and tongue. It is made up of cartilage, ligaments and muscles, which in a series of movements close the entrance to the larynx during swallowing and ensure that food passes into the oesophagus, thereby preventing aspiration.

Trachea (windpipe)

The trachea consists of 16–20 C-shaped cartilage rings. They are joined at the back by connective tissue and involuntary muscle. This design allows for maximum support and patency of the trachea so that it does not collapse inspiration. The mucociliary escalator continues to work within this Nerve endings within the trachea, larynx and bronchioles are sensitive and enable a powerful cough reflex to be initiated as a protective mechanism.

Bronchi and bronchioles

The trachea then bifurcates (splits in two) into the right and left main bronchi at a point called the carina. This is the anatomical position at which the upper respiratory tract becomes the lower respiratory tract. This area has a sensitive cough reflex. The length of an adult bronchus is 12–15 cm. Once inside the lungs the primary bronchus divides on each side until there are 23 divisions in total. Bronchioles are small bronchi with a diameter of less than 1 mm. They can be occluded by mucus, oedema and muscle wall contraction. As the bronchi become smaller the amount of cilia and cartilage reduces whilst smooth muscle increases. This region is innervated by the autonomic nervous system (ANS). When the sympathetic division of the ANS increases its activity it releases hormones, such as epinephrine, which relax smooth muscle. This results in the dilatation of the bronchioles, and therefore more air is able to enter the lungs during inspiration.

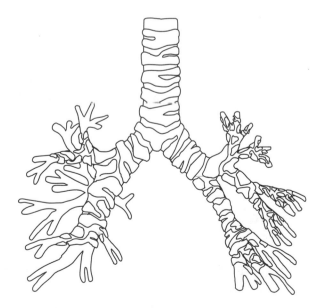

Figure 1.2 Bronchi and bronchioles.

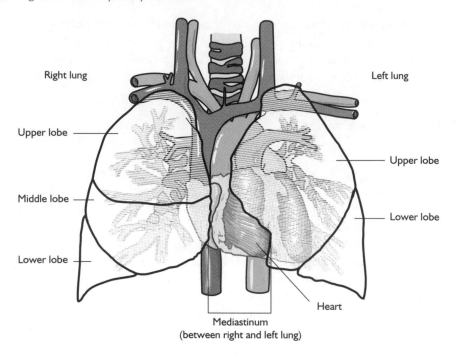

Right lung

Left lung

Upper lobe

Upper lobe

Middle lobe

Lower lobe

Lower lobe

Heart

Mediastinum
(between right and left lung)

Figure 1.3 The lungs.

Lung and pleura

The right lung is divided into three lobes: upper, middle and lower. The left lung, on the other hand, is smaller and has only two lobes (upper and lower) due to the position of the heart.

Each lung has a pleura, which is a continuous serous membrane. The visceral pleura lines the lung, whilst the parietal pleura lines the thoracic cavity. The potential space between them is called the pleural cavity or intrapleural space. It is filled with a fine layer of serous liquid that allows the pleura to glide across each other during inspiration and expiration.

Respiratory zone

This is the part of the respiratory system involved in gaseous exchange.

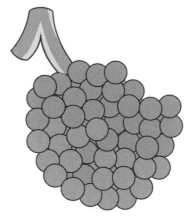

Figure 1.4 Alveoli.

Respiratory bronchioles and alveoli

Alveoli are spherical in shape. There are 300–500 million alveoli in the lungs, the combined surface area of which is approximately the size of a tennis court – between 50 and 100 m^2. This large area of single-layered cells is excellent for gaseous exchange. Two types of epithelial cell are present in the alveoli: Type 1 cells (alveolar cells) are squamous epithelium and form nearly all the network of capillaries; Type 2 cells (septal cells) produce a substance called surfactant. It is a complex mixture of phospholipids and lipoproteins and is essential for increasing lung compliance by reducing surface tension and preventing alveolar collapse. High lung compliance means that the lungs can stretch easily.

The cycle of breathing occurs approximately 12–16 times per minute. During inspiration the 11 pairs of external intercostal muscles that lie between the ribs contract and cause the ribs to move upwards and outwards like bucket handles. Other muscles that raise the rib cage are the sternocleidomastoids, which lift the sternum; the anterior serrati, which lift the ribs; and the scaleni, which lift the first two ribs. The main muscle of breathing, called the diaphragm, is dome-shaped and moves downwards during inspiration. This means that the surface area within the thoracic cavity increases and the pressure therefore decreases relative to atmospheric pressure. The resulting pressure gradient causes air to be sucked into the thorax.

Expiration, on the other hand, is largely a passive process in the healthy individual and occurs when the intercostal muscles and diaphragm relax. Other muscles that pull the rib cage down during expiration are the abdominal recti and internal intercostal muscles.

5

Control of breathing

Hypoventilation (under-breathing) or hyperventilation (over-breathing) can be influenced by physiological, chemical and emotional causes.

The basic control of breathing is performed by the respiratory centres of the brainstem in the medulla and pons. Within the medulla oblongata there are the dorsal respiratory group (DRG) and the ventral respiratory group (VRG). When the neurones from the DRG are activated they travel along the phrenic nerve (which controls the diaphragm) and the intercostal nerve (which controls the external intercostal muscles). This causes them to contract, resulting in the thorax expanding, and inspiration occurs. The DRG then becomes inactive and expiration occurs passively due to elastic recoil of the lungs and muscular relaxation. The activity of the VRG is not clear, but it possesses neurones which connect the medulla to the spinal cord, which are thought to influence forced breathing.

The pons consists of two areas called the pneumotaxic and the apneustic centres. The pneumotaxic centre prevents over-inflation of the lung by transmitting impulses which inhibit inspiration. The apneustic centre prolongs inspiration.

Chemoreceptors

Central chemoreceptors are located in a part of the brainstem called the medulla and are more sensitive to changes in CO_2 than peripheral chemoreceptors. They respond to the concentration of hydrogen ions within the cerebrospinal fluid. The blood–brain barrier does not allow ions to diffuse across it, but carbon dioxide does. When carbon dioxide enters the cerebrospinal fluid it results in an increase of free hydrogen ions which then activate the central chemoreceptors; these in turn stimulate the respiratory centres. Increasing the rate of breathing allows carbon dioxide to be breathed out, resulting in lower levels within the body.

Arterial partial pressure of oxygen (PaO_2) is maintained by peripheral chemoreceptors. These are aortic bodies situated in the aortic arch and carotid bodies positioned around the carotid sinus. They are sensitive to changes in temperature, blood flow, blood pH, pressure of arterial oxygen and carbon dioxide.

Oxygen and carbon dioxide transport

Oxygen is carried in two ways by the blood. Most is carried combined with haemoglobin, but a small amount is dissolved in the plasma. Haemoglobin is a pigment containing the iron part (haem) and a protein (globulin).

Each haemoglobin molecule contains an iron atom that can bind to up to four oxygen molecules. Therefore one haemoglobin molecule is capable of carrying four oxygen molecules when fully saturated. Haemoglobin can load and unload oxygen molecules one at a time and can therefore exist as Hb (unsaturated) HbO_2, HbO_4, HbO_6 or HbO_8, which is fully saturated. This is why the oxygen dissociation curve is sigma- (S-) shaped. Once one oxygen molecule is attached to the haemoglobin its ability to attach more is increased.

Carbon dioxide is carried in three ways. A small amount (7–10%) is dissolved in plasma. Twenty per cent is chemically bound to haemoglobin and carried in the red blood cells. The largest amount (70%) is transported as bicarbonate ion in the plasma. Carbon dioxide combines with water to from carbonic acid, but is quickly dissociated into hydrogen and bicarbonate. It is summarised as the following reversible chemical equation

$$CO_2 + H_2O \rightarrow H_2CO_3 \rightarrow H^+ + HCO3^-$$

Ventilation/perfusion (VQ)

The perfect situation within the lung would be where all of the lung tissue received equal amounts of alveolar ventilation and the pulmonary capillaries that surround the alveoli received an equal amount of the cardiac output. In this case ventilation and perfusion would be matched. However, the reality is that, even for healthy lungs, ventilation/perfusion mismatch occurs. The upper zones of the lung are often over-ventilated whilst the lower zones are comparatively over-perfused but under-ventilated. When a VQ mismatch arises in a diseased lung, shunting can occur. This means that some blood reaches the arterial system without being ventilated. The result of this is that the shunted blood resembles venous blood. Oxygen levels will be low and carbon dioxide levels will be high. Pulmonary blood vessels have the ability to constrict if localised hypoxia occurs. This diverts blood from poorly ventilated to well-ventilated areas.

Pulmonary circulation

The lungs receive blood from pulmonary and bronchial arteries. Deoxygenated blood enters the pulmonary trunk emerging from the right ventricle and divides into the pulmonary arteries – the right pulmonary artery entering the right lung and the left pulmonary artery into the left lung. (The pulmonary arteries are the only arteries to carry deoxygenated blood.) The blood then passes through the arterioles and into smaller capillaries.

Oxygen diffuses from high pressure in the alveoli to lower pressure of the blood. The diffusion continues until the pressure of oxygen in the capillary is equal to that in the alveoli. The blood is now oxygenated. It then flows out in the capillaries through venules to the heart via the pulmonary veins that drain into the left atrium. Bronchial arteries arise from the aorta and take oxygenated blood to the lungs, allowing perfusion via the bronchi and bronchial walls.

Respiratory volumes and capacities

The cycle of respiration occurs on average 12 times per minute. Each breath moves approximately 500 ml of air (tidal voume). Therefore the amount of air moved in one minute = 12 × 500 ml = 6000 ml. This is the minute ventilation rate. A lower than normal minute ventilation rate is a sign of pulmonary malfunction. The equipment used to record the volume of air exchanged during breathing is called a spirometer. Below are the expected normal values for a healthy adult male.

- **Tidal volume**
Amount of air inhaled and exhaled in one breath at rest = 500 ml

- **Inspiratory reserve volume**
The amount of air that can be forcibly inspired beyond the tidal volume = 3000 ml

- **Expiratory reserve volume**
The amount of air that can be forcibly expired beyond the tidal volume = 1100 ml

- **Residual volume**
The air still remaining in the lungs after forced expiration = 1200 ml. This keeps the alveoli inflated.

- **Respiratory capacity**
This involves two more volumes.

  - **Inspiratory capacity**
  Total amount of air that can be inspired after tidal expiration, or

  Inspiratory reserve volume + Tidal volume = 3000 ml + 500 ml

– **Functional residual capacity**
The air remaining in the lungs after tidal expiration, or

Expiratory reserve volume + Residual volume = 1100 ml + 1200 ml

■ **Vital capacity**
The total amount of exchangeable air, or

Expiratory reserve volume + Inspiratory reserve volume + Tidal volume
= 1100 ml + 3000 ml + 500 ml

Dead space refers to the inspired air that fills the conducting system and is not involved in gas exchange.

Practical points

■ Understanding the basic anatomy and physiology of the lungs helps in our understanding of the actual disease process.
■ By understanding what goes wrong with the lungs' normal functioning, the symptoms of many of the lung diseases are more readily explained.

References

Bourke, S. J. (2003) *Respiratory Medicine*, 6th edn. Blackwell Publishing, Oxford.

Guyton, A. and Hall, J. (2006) *Textbook of Medical Physiology*, 11th edn. Elsevier Saunders, Philadelphia.

Jeffries, A. and Turley, A. (1999) *Respiratory System*, Mosby, London.

Law, R. and Bukwirwa, H. (1999) The physiology of oxygen delivery. *Update in Anaesthesia*, **10**, 3.

Marieb, E. (1999) *Human Anatomy and Physiology*, 5th edn. Benjamin Cummings, San Francisco.

Roberts, F. (2000) Respiratory physiology. *Update in Anaesthesia*, **12**, 11.

Tortura, G. and Derrickson, B. (2006) *Principles of Anatomy and Physiology*, 11th edn. John Wiley & Sons, New Jersey.

Waugh, A. and Grant, A. (2001) *Ross and Wilson – Anatomy and Physiology in Health and Illness*, 9th edn. Churchill Livingstone, Edinburgh.

West, J. B. (1998) *Pulmonary Path Physiology – The Essentials*, 5th edn. Lippincott Williams & Wilkins, Philadelphia.

Asthma

Jan Chantrell

Introduction

Asthma is a common and chronic disease that currently affects 5.2 million people in the UK (National Asthma Campaign, 2001). During your career, you will at some point nurse a patient who has a diagnosis of asthma. Patients who have asthma can often get complacent about both their symptoms and their treatment, often not recognising the extent to which asthma is affecting or even controlling what they do in their everyday activities.

The aim of this chapter is to raise your awareness of asthma to allow you to recognise, assess and nurse patients who have asthma more effectively. With only a slight adjustment to treatment, an increase in education or change of device, it is possible to have a high impact on a patient's quality of life. This chapter allows only for an overview of the condition, with some 'must do's' for asthma management and some practical points. There is an array of more detailed literature available at any medical library and in Internet sources. A 'must read' list of sources of information is included at they end of the chapter.

> ## Practical point
>
> If preparing for an assignment involving asthma, narrow your field and look at one aspect of asthma. There are thousands of articles out there!

Definition

The definition of asthma is a very difficult and complex issue. How do you define a disease in which a person can have asthma symptoms triggered by pets and pollens within a particular season but can run the London Marathon, compared to another who is triggered by a fellow passenger on a bus wearing perfume or gets symptoms carrying bags home from a shopping trip? Due to the scope of precipitating factors and variation of symptoms the literature provides an array of definitions. The International Consensus Report (1992) – which is also the definition used by the British Guideline on the Management of Asthma (British Thoracic Society, 2005) – defines asthma as:

> a chronic inflammatory disorder of the airways... in susceptible individuals, inflammatory symptoms are usually associated with widespread but variable airflow obstruction and an increase in airway response to a variety of stimuli. Obstruction is often reversible, either spontaneously or with treatment.

The National Institutes of Health Global Initiative for Asthma (1998) defines asthma as:

> a chronic inflammatory disorder of the airways. In susceptible individuals this inflammation causes recurrent episodes of wheezing, coughing, chest tightness and difficulty in breathing. Inflammation causes airway sensitivity to stimuli such as allergen and irritants...

Practical point

The important message to take from the definitions is that asthma is a chronic inflammatory condition which is variable with regard to onset, symptom severity and stimuli.

Epidemiology

The global prevalence figures for people with asthma have been estimated at between 100 and 150 million (Masoli *et al.*, 2003). In the UK population of

59 million there are over 5 million people receiving treatment for asthma and over 8 million having had a diagnosis of asthma at some point in their lives. A survey of asthma and allergies in childhood (British Thoracic Society, 2006) found that the UK had a 20.7% prevalence rate of asthma in 13–14 year-old children: the fifth highest out of 56 countries worldwide. There are a number of theories thought to contribute to the increase of asthma over the last two decades, and some of these are outlined in Box 2.1.

Box 2.1 Theories associated with increased prevalence of asthma

- Socioeconomic status, e.g. inner city living – pollution, poor ventilation, dampness (Cesaroni et al., 2003).
- Westernised countries – increased hygiene and a sterile environment cause a reduction in microbial exposure, so promoting an atopic status in the very young. This is known as the hygiene hypothesis (Strachan, 2000).
- Dietary intake – over the last 2–3 decades our diets have shifted to include an array of processed and convenience foods at the expense of fresh fruit and vegetables that are high in antioxidants.
- Increased outdoor pollution – not only has there been an increase in traffic, but also a change in the fuels used.

Pathophysiology

The pathophysiology of asthma is very complex. Research is continually identifying further cells and mediators involved with the mechanism of asthma. As previously stated, asthma is a chronic inflammatory disorder. Inflammation is the underlying feature that can cause many pathological changes in the airway (see Table 2.1 and Figure 2.1).

It is often useful to discuss the basic pathophysiology with our patients. Knowledge increases understanding, not only regarding the condition but also the symptoms and treatments. Three possible points to discuss with your patients may be (Figure 2.3):

Table 2.1 Pathological changes in asthma.

Mucus plugging can cause narrowing or occlusion of airway	Epithelial goblet cells are responsible for producing mucus in the airway. These cells can proliferate rapidly, producing large amounts of mucus. This mucus can then trap debris from damaged or shredding epithelial cells. The mucus is usually white or yellow in appearance (see Figure 2.2).
	An increase of mucus production and leakage of fluid from the surrounding tissues can be caused by inflammatory mediators (see Table 2.2) that lead to mucosal oedema.
Epithelial shredding	Epithelium cells can be shredded or damaged. These cells can then not only add to the burden of mucus in the lumen but also: ■ expose the airway by loss of the protective barrier ■ expose nerve fibres ■ reduce the level of a relaxant mediator normally produced by the epithelium cells
Airway remodelling	In chronic asthma structural changes such as: ■ thickening of the collagen layer in subepithelial tissue and basement membranes ■ smooth muscle hypotrophy and hyperplasia
Airway hyper-responsiveness	Smooth muscle in the airway is hyper-reactive to various stimuli. This results in narrowing of the airways. The pathological changes described above can contribute to airway hyper-responsiveness.

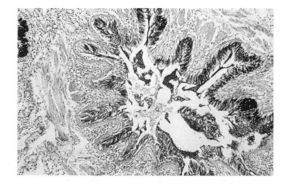

Figure 2.1 Pathological changes in asthma.

Table 2.2 Cells and mediators involved in inflammation.

Inflammatory cells involved in inflammation:	Inflammatory mediators involved in inflammation:
■ Eosinophils ■ Macrophages ■ T-lymphocytes ■ Neutrophils ■ Mast cells	■ Histamine ■ Prostaglandins ■ Leukotrienes ■ Platelet-activating factor ■ Cytokines ■ Major basic protein ■ Substance P ■ Enothelins ■ Plus many others

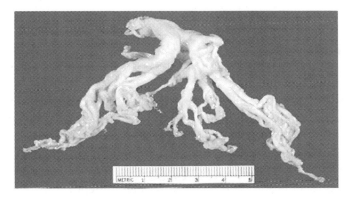

Figure 2.2 Mucus plug.

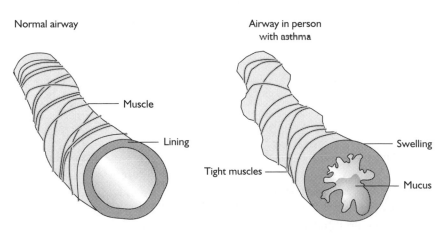

Normal airway

Airway in person with asthma

Muscle

Lining

Tight muscles

Swelling

Mucus

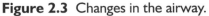

Figure 2.3 Changes in the airway.

1. Inflammation affects the lining of the airways.
2. Muscle around the airway becomes tight, narrowing the space that is used to breathe through.
3. Mucus and debris can be increased – which can lodge in the airway, again adding to the narrowing of the airway.

Practical Point

When reading about pathophysiology of asthma, ensure your literature is up to date. This is to ensure that the content contains all the new research.

Diagnosis of asthma

The diagnosis of asthma can be very difficult due to individual triggers and symptom expression. Initially the diagnosis is made purely by the clinical history, and sometimes – particularly in primary care – this remains the most significant diagnosing feature. The investigations and objective tests are often used as a means to confirm an asthma diagnosis. As you can imagine, ensuring that the correct questions are asked within an in-depth clinical history is of paramount importance to establish the diagnosis (see Box 2.2).

The first step with the clinical history is to establish what the presenting symptoms are, when they occur and if the patient is aware of any precipitating factors. The symptoms patients present with can be one, all, or a combination of the following:

- Wheezing
- Shortness of breath
- Cough
- Chest tightness

The symptoms will be variable, intermittent, often worse at night and provoked by a variety of triggers and irritants (see Figure 2.4). It is important to recognise the presentation of these symptoms, as they are also prominent features of other respiratory diseases, such as COPD, bronchiectasis, cystic fibrosis or even an inhaled foreign body.

Box 2.2 History required to establish an asthma diagnosis

1. Past medical history?
2. Past atopic medical history, e.g. eczema, rhinitis?
3. Family history?
4. Occupation/hobbies/interests?
5. Current or ex-smoker? If yes, how many per day and for how many years?
6. What are the presenting symptoms?
7. When do the symptoms occur, e.g. morning/evening? (Any diurnal variation?)
8. Any seasonal variation to the symptoms?
9. What is the severity of the symptoms, e.g. any admissions to hospital/number of courses of oral steroids per year?
10. Any known triggers, e.g. pets, pollens, exercise, medication?
11. Previous medication, either prescription or over the counter?
12. Was the medication effective?

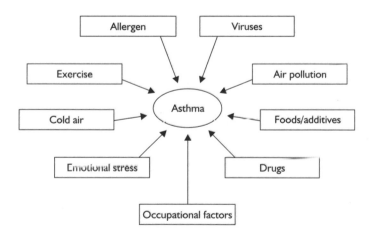

Figure 2.4 Common asthma triggers and irritants.

If the history indicates a clinical suspicion of asthma you might wish to perform an investigation or objective test to confirm the diagnosis. Asthma is a condition which is known as an obstructive airways disease, so many of the tests look at the obstructive element of breathing and the reversal of that obstruction when treatment is given. If you look back at the pathophysiology of asthma you will see that most of the aspects are concerned with blocking or obstructing the airway.

Peak flow measurements

One of the most common tests to identify obstruction is a peak flow measurement (see Figure 2.5). A peak flow recording is a very simple test that can be performed in hospital, at the practice or within the patient's home to measure obstruction. To establish a diagnosis the patient will need to record two weeks of peak flow measurements. These measurements are performed twice a day, morning and early evening. On average, a person's peak flow measurement is worse in the early morning, with the best recording achievable by midday. However, with work or school commitments early evening is adequate. The twice daily recordings will show whether there has been any diurnal variation. Diurnal variation means a difference between the morning and evening recordings (see Figure 2.6). For patients that do not have asthma, or if their asthma is well controlled, the diurnal variation is around 5% (Higgins *et al.*, 1989). To confirm a diagnosis of asthma you are looking for a diurnal variation of around 20% for three days per week in at least two consecutive weeks (British Thoracic Society, 2005). An individual isolated measurement of peak flow will not be indicative of asthma. An isolated peak flow recording is only useful if you have previously established the individual patient's predicted or best peak flow measurement. A predicted peak flow measurement is calculated by age, sex and ethnic origin. If a patient has a high level of physical fitness, or is a singer or musician, this can increase the individual patient's peak flow capability. Once a patient has been diagnosed

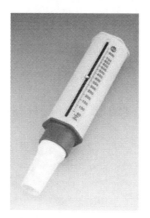

Figure 2.5 Peak flow meter.

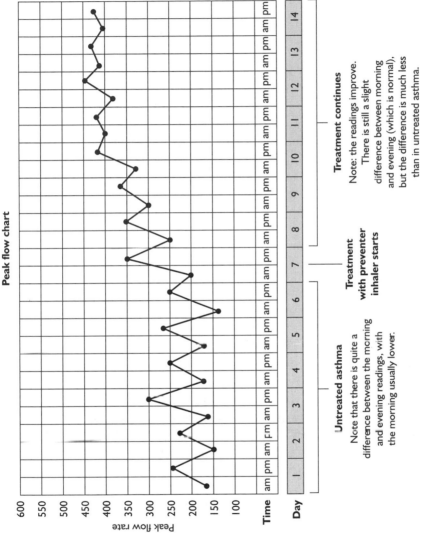

Peak flow chart

Peak flow rate: 600, 550, 500, 450, 400, 350, 300, 250, 200, 150, 100

Time: am pm am pm am pm am pm am pm am pm am pm am pm am pm am pm am pm am pm am pm am pm

Day: 1 2 3 4 5 6 7 8 9 10 11 12 13 14

Untreated asthma
Note that there is quite a difference between the morning and evening readings, with the morning usually lower.

Treatment with preventer inhaler starts

Treatment continues
Note: the readings improve. There is still a slight difference between morning and evening (which is normal), but the difference is much less than in untreated asthma.

Figure 2.6 Serial peak flow recording showing diurnal variation.

with asthma, establishing the patient's best peak flow will help the patient to recognise deteriorating asthma – the peak flow measurements will fall, enabling the patient to either initiate further treatment or seek medical help. This is known as self-management.

Spirometry

Spirometry is a breathing test which can measure levels and severity of obstruction within the airway. This procedure his been used within secondary care for many years, but is now becoming common practice within primary care since the introduction of disease registers for chronic illness (British Medical Association, 2003). Measurements are made of the patient's forced expiratory volume in one second (FEV_1) and the forced vital capacity (FVC). This means how much air a patient can expel under force in one second compared to the total amount of air that the patient's airways are capable of holding. The severity of obstruction can then be measured – large unobstructed airways will expel more air quicker than narrow obstructed airways. The narrower or more obstructed the airway the less breath can be expelled in one second compared with the total amount of breath contained within the airway.

Reversibility

Asthma is known as a reversible airways disease. Testing whether the obstruction within the airway is reversible will help to confirm an asthma diagnosis. Reversibility is simple to perform, but bronchdilators need to be avoided for a number of hours preceding the test, which can prove difficult for some patients. The test is performed by initially recording the patient's peak flow or spirometry. A bronchodilator (e.g. salbutamol or terbutaline) is then prescribed either by an inhaler device (usually a metered dose inhaler and spacer) or nebuliser. Fifteen minutes following the medication either the peak flow or spirometry is repeated. If the peak flow shows a 20% increase or the spirometery shows a 15% or 200 ml increase this can confirm an asthma diagnosis. It is important to note that if a patient's asthma is currently controlled, or if the precipitating factor is currently avoided (e.g. the test is performed in the winter for grass pollen-induced asthma) there will be little or no reversibility (Tweeddale *et al.*, 1987).

Steroid trial

A steroid trial is often used either to establish asthma in a child who is too young to perform breathing tests (due to inability to understand/perform the test) or in an elderly patient who may have a combination of respiratory illnesses (e.g. COPD and asthma). A steroid trial can be performed in a number of different ways:

- Oral steroid e.g. prednisolone 30–40 mg is prescribed daily for two weeks. A child's dose is calculated by weight and equates to 2 mg per kg per day. To assess effectiveness of the medication either peak flow measurements are recorded twice daily for the two weeks, or spirometry is performed at the beginning and end of the course. An increase of 20% in the peak flow recordings and an increase of 15% or 200 ml will confirm asthma.
- Inhaled steroid therapy e.g. beclometasone, can be used for a steroid trial, but a longer period of time is required to assess the efficacy of the medication, which is usually six weeks. The peak flow is recorded twice daily over the six-week period. Spirometry is performed before and after the six-week period.
- For children unable to perform the peak flow or spirometry tests, a diary is used to record the child's symptoms before, during and after either the inhaled or oral steroids are used.

PC$_{20}$, sputum induction and nitric oxide

PC$_{20}$, sputum induction and nitric oxide tests are currently limited to patients attending secondary care units. However, there has been some work to try to make nitric oxide measurement equipment available within primary care (Smith *et al.*, 2005). Nitric oxide is a gas that is released by inflammatory mediators in the lung and can be measured in expelled breath. A debate regarding how sensitive this test is to establish the severity of asthma continues, with ongoing research (Berry *et al.*, 2005).

A PC$_{20}$ test is used to diagnose hyper-reactivity within the airway when there are minimal symptoms or to refute a previous asthma diagnosis (e.g. a patient wishing to join the armed forces but who has a record of asthma as a very young child). A PC$_{20}$ test is performed by nebulising either histamine or methocholine solution to induce bronchoconstriction. These substances, if given in sufficient quantities, will induce bronchoconstriction in any individual, with or without asthma. The PC$_{20}$ test initially uses dilute concentrations of either methocholine or histamine, with approximately eight incremental doses. The highest concentration is 16 mg. Spirometry is recorded as a baseline and after each nebulised dose. Once the FEV_1 is reduced by 20% the test is stopped and the preceding dose concentration is recorded. For a 20% reduction in FEV_1 recorded at 8 mg or below, asthma/hyper-reactivity can be diagnosed.

Induced sputum tests are currently being performed within secondary care units. Initially a test purely used in research, it has now been proved to be very useful in the clinical area (Green *et al.*, 2002). The sputum is induced by the inhalation of nebulised saline. The saline causes the patient to cough and expectorate sputum. Different strengths of saline will allow mucus to be expectorated from different parts of the airway (e.g. large or small airways). Once the sputum has been expectorated from the airway it can be stained, allowing inflammatory cells to be identified and counted (e.g. eosinophils and neutrophils).

Practical Points

- A peak flow measurement is patient effort-dependent. If a patient cannot perform the test with adequate effort the test is null and void.
- If a patient's asthma is currently well controlled (i.e. no symptoms, little or no reliever (bronchodilator) usage, or no trigger exposure, e.g. outside the pollen season), the peak flow will not show diurnal variation of 20%.
- Correct technique and consistent patient effort are required to perform both peak flow and spirometry measurements.
- You will find more details about spirometry in Chapter 5 (on COPD).
- Understanding and interpretation of the recordings is essential for the healthcare professional.
- Sputum induction is done by nebulising salt water; this tastes horrible and is not a pleasant experience for the patient.

Treatment of asthma

Current treatment and management of asthma in the UK follows the guidelines produced by the British Thoracic Society and Scottish Intercollegiate Network

(British Thoracic Society, 2005). The aim of asthma treatment is to control symptoms and minimise exacerbations. Asthma fatality figures for 2004 inclusive of all ages are 1,381 (British Thoracic Society, 2006) and there remains no cure for asthma. The British Thoracic Society (2005) has produced guidelines in the form of a stepwise approach to asthma treatment. The aim of the stepwise approach offered by the guideline is to manage the variability of asthma symptoms, allowing treatment to be either 'stepped up' or 'stepped down' as appropriate. For example, if a patient were to be admitted onto a respiratory or medical ward with severe symptoms of asthma, the treatment that they would receive might well be that which is listed in step 4 of the guidelines. However, as the patient is stabilised the treatment reduces and the patient moves down the steps. Another example would be a patient normally requiring bronchodilator treatment infrequently (twice a month) to daily. This patient would then require an increase of treatment (inhaled steroid) and move to step 2 of the guidelines.

As you can see, there are a number of different medications used to treat asthma. Most asthma medication is administered by inhalation. This allows for direct action within the airway, allowing for reduced doses of medication and a reduction in systemic side effects. The most common medications are described below.

Beta₂ agonists

Beta$_2$ agonists are also known as relievers or bronchodilators (see Table 2.3). Beta$_2$ agonists stimulate the B$_2$-adrenergic receptors in bronchial smooth muscle, enhance mucociliary clearance and decrease vascular permeability. Their action usually lasts for four hours and they are usually taken as an 'as required' medication. They can also be taken prior to exercise – whether it is football or making the bed – allowing the patient to perform that activity. Common side-effects include tachycardia, palpitations, tremors and headaches.

Inhaled corticosteroids (steroids)

Inhaled steroids (see Table 2.3) are the mainstay of asthma treatment. They reduce inflammatory cells within the airway, reduce bronchial hyper-reactivity, improve or reduce the rate of decline in lung function and can improve airway remodelling (Laitinen *et al.*, 1992; Pederson *et al.*, 1993; Ward *et al.*, 2002).

Table 2.3 Common inhaler preparations and associated devices.

Drugs – Brand and generic names	Devices – This list gives an overview of devices available. Please see BNF[1] for correct device for each medication.
Beta₂ agonists	
Salbutamol or Ventolin, Aerolin, Aerimir, Asmasal and Salamol	MDI[2], Accuhaler, Dischaler, Auto-haler, Clickhaler, Easibreath and Pulvinal
Terbutaline or Bricanyl	Turbohaler and MDI
Inhaled corticosteroids	
Beclometasone or Becotide, Qvar, Beclazone, Aerobec and Aerobec forte, Asmabec and Filair	MDI, Accuhaler, Dischaler, Auto-haler, Clickhaler, Pulvinal and Easi-breath,
Budesonide or Pulmicort	Turbohaler and Novolizer
Fluticasone or Flixotide	MDI and Accuhaler
Mometasone or Asmanex	Twisthaler
Ciclesonide or Alvesco	MDI
Long-acting beta agonists	
Salmeterol or Serevent	MDI and Accuhaler
Formoterol or Oxis	Turbohaler
	Spacers – Common spacers include Volumatic, Aerochamber plus, Able Spacer, Nebuhaler

[1]BNF – *British National Formulary*
[2]MDI – Metered dose inhaler

   Inhaled steroids are a long-term treatment, generally taken twice daily with or without asthma symptoms. They take at least two weeks for the patient to notice any improvement, with maximum benefit occurring at around three months (Laitinen *et al.*, 1992). It is common for patients not to understand the different effects of inhaled steroids and beta₂ agonists within the airway. The beta agonist improves symptoms of breathlessness within a few moments, but the effect of inhaled steroids is not so obvious. If we are expecting patients to use a medication twice daily, even when asymptomatic, for a prolonged period of time, it is essential to discuss the mechanisms and possible side-effects with the patient. The common side-effects of inhaled steroids are local and caused by deposition on the mouth and pharynx. They include hoarseness of the voice, candidiasis (thrush) of the throat and/or mouth, soreness and/or irritation of the throat and coughing. There are also rare systemic side-effects occurring after long-term use of high doses of inhaled steroids, e.g. suppression of the production of adrenocorticotrophic hormone (ACTH), changes to bone metabolism, a reduction of skin thickness and an increase of cataracts in adult patients. There are a number of measures to reduce these possible side-effects, which include:

- Ensure that the minimum/lowest dose of inhaled steroids is prescribed
- Use spacer devices
- Rinse mouth following inhalation of therapy
- Change to an alternative inhaled steroid
- Advice regarding diet and exercise to encourage good bone growth
- Be aware of total steroid use, e.g. nasal sprays, topical steroid creams
- For high dose inhaled corticosteroids a steroid warning card should be given to the patient

Long-acting Beta$_2$ agonists (LABA)

Over the last decade long-acting Beta$_2$ agonists (LABA) have become a prominent feature at step 3 of the British Thoracic Society (2005) Guidelines in the management of asthma. LABA not only relax smooth muscle cells in the airway for a period of 12 hours but also may potentiate the effects of inhaled steroids (Greening *et al.*, 1994; Woolcock *et al.*, 1996; Pauwels *et al.*, 1997). The side-effects most commonly associated with LABA are similar to those of Beta$_2$ agonists and comprise tremor, palpitations and headache. The medications are required twice daily in conjunction with inhaled steroids and there have been a small number of combination therapies produced, e.g. Seretide (fluticasone and salmeterol) and Symbicort (budesonide and formeterol).

Leukotriene receptor antagonists

Leukotriene receptor antagonists (LTRA) reduce asthma symptoms not only by inhibiting the bronchoconstrictor effects of leukotrienes, but also by anti-inflammatory effects that can result in clinical improvement within 24 hours. Both inhaled steroids and oral steroids are unable to inhibit the increased leukotriene production in asthma, but it remains unclear the extent to which anti-leukotriene therapy can reduce inflammation in the same way as inhaled steroids. Some patients respond dramatically to LTRA, while others have a lesser response. Although patients may notice an improvement in symptoms within

24 hours, it is recommended that a trial of treatment continue for a period of 6 weeks. Side-effects associated with LTRA consist of headaches, sore throat and (rarely) changes in liver enzymes.

Theophylline

The mechanism by which theophylline works is unclear. It does have bronchodilator effects and may influence the influx and activity of inflammatory cells. Theophylline is used in the UK at either step 4 or 5 of the British Thoracic Society (2005) Guidelines or can be used intravenously in the treatment of acute asthma exacerbations within secondary care, as cardiac monitoring and full resuscitation facilities need to be available. Theophylline is given orally and has a narrow therapeutic range. A plasma theophylline concentration of 20 mg/L is required for optimum bronchodilation. If higher concentrations are maintained the risk of side-effects from is increased. Common side-effects are nausea, vomiting, tachycardia, arrhythmias, insomnia, seizures and sudden death.

Oral corticosteroids (steroids)

Oral steroids are reserved for patients who are unable to control symptoms on maximum inhaled therapy (step 4 of the British Thoracic Society (2005)

Practical points

- If you are nursing a patient taking theophylline ensure that you read the drug interactions section carefully in the BNF.
- Always check inhaler technique at every opportunity.
- Discuss with your patients how they are copying with taking regular medications. Do they know what all their inhalers are for and when they should be taking them?
- There are other medications that can be given for the treatment of asthma, such as oxygen, cromones and ipratropium bromide or other treatments that are given alongside asthma medications such as antibiotics and antihistamines.
- Try to obtain some placebo inhalers and have a go yourself at the different techniques required to deliver the medication to the airway. It's a bit like riding a bike – it looks easy enough until you have a go.

Guidelines) or who have acute, severe or life-threatening exacerbations of asthma. The side-effects previously discussed in the inhaled steroid section become more of a risk if receiving long-term oral steroids (step 5 of the Guidelines). When oral steroids are given for an acute exacerbation it is important to ensure that the patient's symptoms and peak flow have returned to normal before stopping or tapering the dose. If a patient has received less than 21 days of oral steroid to regain control, no tapering is required. If, however, the course is longer than 21 days or if the course is repeated within six weeks of a previous course, tapering is required. Tapering the dose will depend on how long the patient has been taking oral steroids and may vary from 5 mg daily to 5 mg weekly to 1 mg every two to four weeks.

Education

As we have previously discussed in this chapter, asthma is a chronic and variable condition. It can present in different forms of severity and has many different triggers that depend upon the individual's atopic status. As with all chronic diseases, education is very important in all aspects of management. Throughout this chapter certain aspects have been highlighted for discussion with the patient, including the changes in the airway, different medications and their effects within the lung. Patients are individuals and so is their asthma. Patients' health beliefs and psychosocial aspects, as well as particular trigger factors, do not allow identical management of patients with asthma. Communication and discussion regarding what the individual patient wants or needs from their asthma management is always the best place to start. Any patient given frequent or continuous steroids should receive a steroid warning card and prophylaxis against osteoporosis.

Practical points

- A discussion with a patient about what having asthma means to them can often highlight issues you hadn't previously thought about.
- Always check and review inhaler techniques.
- Instead of asking a patient how often they take their steroid inhaler, you may obtain a more accurate picture of concordance by asking them how often they forget their inhaler? This offers acceptance of not taking their medication every day. How often do you complete a course of antibiotics?

By educating patients you are empowering them to take more control of their asthma. Being aware of worsening symptoms of asthma, what their normal or best peak flow is and then having a plan of action of what to do about it can not only improve quality of life but also reduce hospital admissions (Thoonen *et al.*, 2003). There is an array of Action Plans that can be used to help patients recognise and act upon worsening symptoms of asthma. It may be that you don't have access to specific plans, but a simple discussion, followed by a written list of worsening symptoms, may help to prevent a more severe exacerbation in the future.

'Must read' list

British Guideline on the Management of Asthma (see reference list – British Thoracic Society, 2005)
The Burden of Lung Disease (see reference list – British Thoracic Society, 2006).
Asthma: Your Questions Answered, by Antony Crockett. Churchill Livingstone, Edinburgh.
MIMS for Nurses. A practical handbook. Haymarket Publications, London.
GINA (Global Initiative for Asthma) Guidelines – http://www.ginasthma.com/
National Asthma Campaigns website – http://www.asthma.org.uk/
Good site for student healthcare professions – http://www.asthmaexplained.co.uk/
Good site for references – http://www.asthmatool.com/

References

Berry, M., Hargadon, B. and Morgan, A. (2005) Alveola nitric oxide in adults with asthma: evidence of distal lung inflammation in refractory asthma. *European Respiratory Journal*, **25**, 986–91.

British Medical Association (2003) *GMS Contract. Investing in Clinical Practice*. The NHS Confederation. Available at http://www.bma.org.uk/ap.nsf/Content/NewGMSContract/

British Thoracic Society (2005) *British Guideline on the Management of Asthma: a National Clinical Guideline*, rev. edn, November. http//www.brit-thoracic.org.uk/. SIGN Guideline No. 63.

British Thoracic Society (2006) *The Burden of Lung Disease*, 2nd Edition. Available from http://www.brit-thoracic.org.uk/.

Cesaroni, G., Farchi, S., Davoli, M., Forastiere, F. and Perucci, C. (2003) Individual and area-based indicators of socioeconomic status and childhood asthma. *European Respiratory Journal*, **22**, 619–24.

Global Initiative for Asthma (1998) *Asthma Management and Prevention: A Practical Guide for Health Care Professionals*. US Department of Health and Human Studies, Public Health Service & National Heart, Lung and Blood Institute. National Institutes of Health.

Green, R., Brightling, C., McKenna, S., Hargadon, B., Parker, D., Bradding, P., Wardlaw, A. and Pavord. I. (2002) Asthma exacerbations and sputum eosinophil counts: a randomized controlled trial. *Lancet*, **360**, 1715–21.

Greening, A., Ind, P., Northfield, M. and Shaw, G. (1994). Added salmeterol versus higher-dose corticosteroid in asthma patients with symptoms on existing inhaled steroids. *Lancet*, **334**, 219–24.

Higgins, B. G., Britton, J. R. and Chinn, S. (1989) The distribution of peak flow variability in a population sample. *American Review of Respiratory Disease*. **140**, 1368–72.

International Consensus Report on the diagnosis and treatment of asthma (1992) National Heart, Lung and Blood Institute. National Institutes of Health, Bethesda, Maryland. Publication no. 92-3091. *European Respiratory Journal*, 5 March, 601–41.

Laitinen, L., Laitinen, A. and Haahtela, T. (1992) A comparative study of the effects of an inhaled corticosteriod, budesonide and of a B_2 agonist, terbutaline on airway inflammation in newly diagnosed asthmatics. *Journal of Allergy and Clinical Immunology*, **90**, 32–4.

Masoli, M., Fabian, D., Holt, S. and Beasley, R. (2003) *Global Burden of Asthma*. Global Initiative for Asthma.

National Asthma Campaign (2001) *National Asthma Audit*. National Asthma Campaign, London.

Pauwels, R., Lofdahl, C. G. and Postma, D. (1997). Formoterol and Corticosteroid Establishing Therapy (FACET) International Study Group. Effects of inhaled formoterol and budesonide on exacerbations of asthma. *New England Journal of Medicine*, **337**, 1405–11.

Pederson, S. and Agertoft, L. (1993). Effects of long-term budesonide treatment on growth, weight and lung function in children. *American Review of Respiratory Disease*, **147**, 265.

Smith, A. D., Cowan, J. O. and Brassett, K. P. (2005) Use of exhaled nitric oxide measurements to guide treatment in chronic asthma. *New England Journal of Medicine*, **352**, 2163–73.

Strachan, D. (2000) Family size, infection and atopy: the first decade of the 'hygiene hypothesis'. *Thorax*, **55**, S2–10.

Thoonen, B. P., Schermer, T. V. and Van den Boom G. (2003) Self-management of asthma in general practice, asthma control and quality of life: a randomized control trial. *Thorax*, **58**(1), 30–6.

Tweeddale, P. M., Alexander, F. and McHardy, G. J. (1987) Short-term variability of FEV_1 and bronchodilator responsiveness in patients with obstructive ventilatory defects. *Thorax*, **42**, 487–90.

Ward, C., Pavi, M. and Bish, R. (2002) Airway inflammation, basement membrane thickening and bronchial hyper-responsiveness in asthma. *Thorax*, **57**, 309–16.

Woolcock, A., Lundback, B., Ringdal, N. and Jaques, L. A. (1996) Comparison of the addition of salmeterol to inhaled steroids with doubling of the dose of inhaled steroids. *American Journal of Respiratory Critical Care*, **153**, 1481–8.

CHAPTER 3

Bronchiectasis

Karen Payne

Introduction

Bronchiectasis is a permanent abnormal dilation occurring in one or more of the bronchi of the lungs, the cause of which is often hard to determine. In health the air passages produce small amounts of clear mucus; this is swept along by small hair-like structures (cilia) that line the airways. This mucus is then swallowed, generally without us being aware of it. In bronchiectasis this mucociliary clearance mechanism is impaired. The cilia are damaged by chronic bacterial infection and do not clear mucus effectively. As a result of this, extra mucus tends to collect in the parts of the airways that are dilated, and this in turn makes the person more prone to infection and inflammation, leading to progressive damage. Bronchiectasis can be widespread throughout the lungs or confined to a lobe or lobes.

Epidemiology

The epidemiology of bronchiectasis is a reflection of the incidence and prevalence of the causative conditions. The precise incidence of bronchiectasis is uncertain, and it varies greatly depending on the populations studied and the methods used to make the diagnosis (Spencer, 2005). However, severe bronchiectasis is less common in developed countries. This is most likely related to improvements in socioeconomic conditions, childhood immunisation and effective antibiotic therapy for infections (Sapey and Stockley, 2004).

Table 3.1 Age range of patients hospitalised with bronchiectasis.

Age	Percentage
15 to 59 years old	37
60 to 74 years old	41
Over 75 years old	22

In the UK the *Hospital Episodes Statistics for 2003–2004* (Department of Health, 2005) showed that bronchiectasis accounted for 55,648 bed days, approximately 1 in 180 hospital admissions. These statistics also showed that 61% of hospital consultant episodes for bronchiectasis were for women, indicating that there is a female predominance. The average age of patients hospitalised for bronchiectasis was 60 years old. Table 3.1 shows the age range of patients hospitalised with bronchiectasis (Department of Health, 2005).

A recent study of non-cystic fibrosis bronchiectasis in childhood in the UK (Eastham *et al.*, 2005) found a 10-fold higher rate than that of a previous one by Nikolaizik and Warner (1994), felt to be largely due to the introduction of high-resolution computerised tomography to investigate chronic respiratory illness in children, and to some extent a misdiagnosis of asthma in children.

Pathogenesis

Bronchial dilatation is associated with loss of cilia along with vascular changes. These changes are related to chronic bacterial infection and several theories have been put forward to explain this relationship (Spencer, 2005). Perhaps the most widely accepted theory is Cole's (1997), in which he described the pathogenesis of bronchiectasis as a 'vicious circle', where an initial damaging insult to the airways compromises the first-line defence mechanism of the lungs, leading to the start of this circle (Figure 3.1).

1. Impaired mucocilliary clearance leads to the accumulation of secretions.
2. Accumulation of secretions leads to infection by bacteria.
3. Infection by bacteria leads to increased mucus production, resulting in impaired cilliary performance and a greater inflammatory response.
4. Excessive inflammatory response causes tissue damage.
5. Tissue damage eventually produces dilated bronchi, including loss of ciliated epithelium and impaired mucocilliary clearance.
6. Back to step 1.

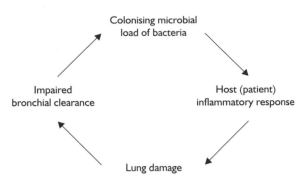

Figure 3.1 The vicious circle of bronchiectasis.

Causes of bronchiectasis

The aetiology of bronchiectasis is unknown in more than half the cases investigated (Cohen and Sahn, 1999). Post-infective bronchial damage (usually in childhood) is the most common identifiable cause in middle-aged and elderly patients. Effective childhood immunisation has led to a marked reduction in the incidence of bronchiectasis caused by infections such as pertussis and measles; however, other childhood respiratory tract infections may contribute to permanent airway damage (Johnston *et al.*, 1998).

Other causes have been identified, such as:

- Primary cilia dyskinesia (PCD) is an inherited condition in which poorly functioning cilia lead to the retention of secretions, causing recurrent infections that in turn lead to bronchiectasis. The estimated frequency of PCD at birth is 1 in 15,000 to 1 in 40,000 (Barker, 2002).
- Tuberculosis (see Chapter 17)
- Cystic fibrosis (see Chapter 4)
- Immunodeficiency syndromes involving deficiencies of IgG, IgM and IgA; Human Immunodeficiency Virus (HIV).
- Obstruction (e.g. foreign body, tumour), which can cause localised bronchiectasis

Pasteur *et al.* (2000) evaluated 150 adults with bronchiectasis to try to establish a cause (Table 3.2). One or more causes were identified in 70 patients (47%), whereas no cause could be established in 80 patients (53%).

Symptoms associated with bronchiectasis are cough, as the patient attempts to clear excess mucus, repeated chest infections and breathlessness. Due to these clinical features of bronchiectasis, there is a misconception that it is

Table 3.2 Causes and associations of bronchiectasis (*n* = 150) (Pasteur *et al.*, 2000).

Cause	n	(%)
Idiopathic	80	53
ABPA[1]	11	7
Immune defect	12	8
Total humoral	11	7
Total neutrophil function	1	
<1 Rheumatoid arthritis	4	3
Ulcerative colitis	2	<1
Cilliary dysfunction	3	1.5
Young's syndrome	5	3
Cystic fibrosis	4	3
Post-infectious	44	29
Aspiration	6	4
Panbronchiolitis	1	<1
Congenital	1	<1

[1]ABPA = allergic bronchopulmonary aspergillosis

caused by smoking, but in fact 80% of patients have never smoked and most of the remainder have stopped (British Lung Foundation, 2004). Those patients continuing to smoke should be advised to stop, as smoking further impairs the mucociliary clearance.

Clinical features

Virtually all patients with bronchiectasis have cough and chronic sputum production. Dyspnoea and wheeze occur in about 75% and chest pain in 50% of patients. One third of patients have signs of chronic sinusitis and nasal polyps (Barker, 2002). Recurrent exacerbations are common, as the mucus-filled inflamed airways make an ideal environment for bacteria to grow and multiply.

Haemoptysis is often a very worrying symptom for the patient, normally caused by the bursting of blood vessels in the lungs during a bout of severe or prolonged coughing. It is a relatively common feature of bronchiectasis, occurring in approximately 50% of patients (Silverman *et al.*, 2003). It can vary from streaks of blood in the sputum to coughing up frank blood; however, life-threatening haemoptysis is rare (Mysliwiec and Pina, 1999).

Diagnosis

Standard chest X-rays may show thickened, dilated bronchi (tram lines), but occasionally X-rays are normal.

The gold standard for the diagnosis of bronchiectasis is a High Resolution Computerised Tomography (HRCT) scan (Silverman *et al*., 2003). In normal lungs the bronchi and adjacent artery appear similar in size; however, in patients with bronchiectasis the dilated bronchi appears larger than the artery, giving the appearance of a ring set with a stone (signet ring sign).

Pulmonary function testing (spirometry) is useful in obtaining a baseline assessment of the patient, as well as allowing an objective determination of the deterioration of a patient's pulmonary function. It often reveals airway obstruction, which is not usually reversible, with a reduced ratio of forced expiratory volume in one second (FEV_1) to forced vital capacity (FVC) (Barker, 2002).

Acute exacerbations of bronchiectasis

All patients with bronchiectasis are at greater risk of respiratory infections. The identification of an exacerbation is fairly complex, as in some patients with bronchiectasis sputum can be chronically purulent. However, in a large study by O'Donnell *et al*. (1998) of 349 adult patients in 23 centres including the UK, an exacerbation was defined as including four of the nine symptoms in Table 3.3.

Treatment and management

Antibiotic therapy

The aim of medical treatment is to treat potential infections and the ensuing inflammation of the airways, and to improve mucociliary clearance (Angrill, 2001)

Table 3.3 Symptoms of exacerbation of bronchiectasis (O'Donnell *et al.*, 1998).

- Change in sputum production
- Increased dyspnoea
- Increased cough
- Temperature >38.0 °C
- Increased wheezing
- Malaise, fatigue, lethargy, or decreased exercise tolerance
- Reduced pulmonary function
- Radiographic changes consistent with a new pulmonary process
- Changes in chest sounds

Antibiotics for infections can be given orally, intravenously or via nebulisation. They can be used individually or in combination, and should be guided by sputum cultures.

Oral antibiotics are routinely used for milder exacerbations, whilst moderate to severe exacerbations may require intravenous antibiotics (administered in hospital or at home). Nebulised antibiotics are mostly used prophylactically for chronic infection.

The most frequent organisms isolated are *Haemophilus influenzae* and *Pseudomonas aeruginosa*. Pasteur *et al.* (2000) found that these were also most commonly associated with persistent colonisation (Table 3.4). However, in some patients no organism is ever isolated, despite the patient having purulent sputum.

Physiotherapy

Physiotherapy for bronchiectasis is aimed primarily at clearing the excess thick sputum which characterises this disease (Thompson *et al.*, 2002). The desired outcome is that the frequency of infective exacerbation is reduced, although there is no published evidence to support this. The goal is to clear the sputum with minimal coughing and effort, thus preventing fatigue, further irritation to the lungs and chest pain.

Physiotherapists teach a variety of different techniques that facilitate chest clearance (Webber and Pryor, 1993). Historically, postural drainage with percussion was the treatment of choice; however, there are now other techniques which have been proven as effective, such as the active cycle of breathing, autogenic drainage, flutter, acapella and positive expiratory pressure (PEP)

Table 3.4 Sputum microbiology – patients with bacteria.

Organism	Isolated	Colonising
	n (%)	*n (%)*
Staphylococcus aureus	21 (14)	11 (7)
Streptococcus pneumoniae	20 (13)	6 (4)
Haemophilus influenzae	52 (35)	26 (17)
Moraxella catarrhalis	30 (20)	13 (9)
Pseudomonas aeruginosa	46 (31)	36 (24)
Coliforms	17 (11)	6 (4)
Aspergillus fumigatus	3 (2)	0 (0)
Other	7 (5)	1 (1)
No organisms isolated	34 (23)	

(Langenderfer, 1998; Thompson *et al.*, 2002; Patterson *et al.*, 2005). These techniques can be performed independently and are more flexible and convenient (Main *et al.*, 2005). The choice of technique is made following a detailed assessment of each patient's presenting symptoms.

As with all patients who have a chronic respiratory illness, shortness of breath, physical deconditioning and urinary incontinence (females), often caused by persistent coughing, are other problems that the physiotherapist can help with.

Inhaled bronchodilators

Bronchodilators (e.g. salbutamol) may be used to give symptomatic relief. Inhaled corticosteroids are sometimes used in bronchiectasis in an attempt to reduce airway inflammation; however, evidence for their efficacy is lacking.

Surgery

The role of surgery in bronchiectasis has declined but not disappeared (Barker, 2002). Patients with localised severe bronchiectasis may be candidates for lung resection if they suffer from frequent acute exacerbations despite medical treatment. Surgery may also be used for major haemoptysis.

Lung transplantation may be considered for severe generalised bronchiectasis (Barlow *et al.*, 2000).

Prognosis

Prognosis varies with the predisposing condition. Although bronchiectasis cannot be cured, in general patients do well if they comply with treatment regimes and practice routine preventative strategies. These include regular physiotherapy, avoiding respiratory irritants (e.g. tobacco) and maintaining immunisations. Prompt antibiotic treatment of any infections also reduces the risk of further lung damage (Kolbe, 2005).

The prognosis for bronchiectasis is poorly researched. Keistinen *et al.* (1997) conducted a study to examine the long-term prognosis of this disease and found that for bronchiectatic patients treated in hospital prognosis was better than that for patients with chronic obstructive pulmonary disease (COPD) but poorer than that of patients with asthma.

Conclusion

Bronchiectasis has long been a Cinderella disease, receiving little funding or research interest (Keistinen, 1997). It is a chronic disease requiring long-term follow-up and requires a great deal of effort from the patient and carers to improve outlook and reduce morbidity.

On reviewing the literature it appears that most researchers agree that the introduction of high-resolution computerised tomography has improved the diagnosis of bronchiectasis. Also, it is unlikely that many of the underlying causes of bronchiectasis will be eradicated in the near future (Spencer, 2005). The emphasis should be placed on the need to improve our understanding

Practical points

- Bronchiectasis may be a missed or misdiagnosis in patients and should be considered in patients with chronic sputum production and frequent infections not responding to treatment
- An HRCT scan may be necessary to confirm diagnosis
- Physiotherapy and prompt treatment of infections are vital components of care
- Intravenous antibiotics can be administered by patients at home to reduce the time spent in hospital and the nurse may have an important role in teaching patients to self manage these.

of this condition and the effectiveness of treatment. Ideally, all patients with bronchiectasis should be reviewed by a respiratory specialist, preferably in the context of a multidisciplinary team (Kolbe, 2005). However, for the majority of patients their General Practitioner in the community can carry out long-term follow-up.

References

Angrill, J., Carlos, A. and Torres, A. (2001) Bronchiectasis (review article). *Current Opinion in Infectious Diseases*, **14**(2), 193–7.

Barker, A. F. (2002) Medical progress: bronchiectasis. *New England Journal of Medicine*, **346**(18), 1383–93.

Barlow, C. W., Robbins, R. C., Moon, M. R., Akkindipe, O., Theodore, J. and Reitz, B. A. (2000) Heart-lung versus double-lung transplantation for suppurative lung disease. *Journal of Thoracic and Cardiovascular Surgery*, **119**, 466–76.

British Lung Foundation (2004) *What is Bronchiectasis?* The Facts Leaflet. British Lung Foundation, London.

Cohen, M. and Sahn, S. A. (1999) Bronchiectasis in systemic diseases. *Chest*, **116**, 1063–74.

Cole, P. (1997) The damaging role of bacteria in chronic lung infection. *Journal of Antimicrobial Chemotherapy*, **40** (suppl. A), 5–10.

Department of Health (2005) *Hospital Episodes Statistics for 2003–2004.* http://www.dh.gov.uk/.

Eastham, K., Fall, A., Mitchell, L. and Spencer, D. A. (2004) The need to redefine non-cystic fibrosis bronchiectasis in childhood. *Thorax*, **59**, 324–7.

Johnston, I. D., Strachan, D. P. and Anderson, H. R. (1998) Effect of pneumonia and whooping cough in childhood on adult lung function. *New England Journal of Medicine*, **338**, 581–7.

Keistinen, T., Saynajakangas, O., Tuuponen, T. and Kivela, S. L. (1997) Bronchiectasis: an orphan disease with a poorly-understood prognosis, *European Respiratory Journal*, **10**, 2784–7.

Kolbe, J. (2005) Bronchiectasis – a Patient's Guide. http://www.medic8.com/.

Langenderfer, B. (1998) Alternatives to percussion and postural drainage. A review of mucus clearance therapies: percussion and postural drainage, autogenic drainage, positive expiratory pressure, flutter valve, intrapulmonary percussive ventilation, and high frequency chest compression with the Thairapy vest. *Journal of Cardiopulmonary Rehabilitation*, **18**(4), 283–9.

Main, E., Prasad, A. and Van der Schans, C. (2005) Conventional chest physiotherapy compared to other airway clearance for cystic fibrosis. *Cochrane Database of Systematic Reviews*, Issue 1.

Mysliwiec, V. and Pina, J. S. (1999) Bronchiectasis: the 'other' obstructive lung disease. *Postgraduate Medicine*, **106**(1), 123–31.

Nikolaizik, W. H. and Warner, J. O. (1994) Aetiology of chronic suppurative lung disease. *Archives of Disease in Childhood*, **70**, 141–2.

O'Donnell, A. E., Barker, A. F., Ilowite, J. S. and Fick, R. B. (1998) Treatment of idiopathic bronchiectasis with aerosolized recombinant human DNase, *Chest*, **113**, 1329–34.

Pasteur, M. C., Helliwell, S. M., Houghton, S. J., Webb, S. J., Foweraker, J. E., Coulden, R. A., Flower, C. D., Bilton, D. and Keogan, M. T. (2000) An investigation into causative factors in patients with bronchiectasis. *American Journal of Respiratory and Critical Care Medicine*, **162**(4), 1277–84.

Patterson, J. E., Bradley, J. M., Hewitt, O., Bradbury, I. and Elborn, S. (2005) Airway clearance in bronchiectasis: a randomised crossover trial of active cycle of breathing techniques versus Acapella. *Respiration*, **72**(3), 239–42.

Sapey, E. and Stockley, R. (2004) Bronchiectasis. *Medicine*, **32**(2), 153–8.

Silverman, E., Ebright, L., Kwiatkowski, M. and Cullina, J. (2003) Current management of bronchiectasis: review and 3 case studies. *Heart and Lung*, **32**(1), 59–64.

Spencer, D. A. (2005) From hemp seed and porcupine quill to HRCT: advances in the diagnosis and epidemiology of bronchiectasis. *Archives of Disease in Childhood*, **90**, 712–14.

Thompson, C. S., Harrison, S., Ashley, J., Day, K. and Smith, D.L. (2002) Randomised crossover study of the flutter device and the active cycle of breathing technique in non-CF bronchiectasis. *Thorax*, **57**(5), 446–8.

Webber, B. A. and Pryor, J. A. (1993) *Physiotherapy for Respiratory and Cardiac Problems*. Churchill Livingstone, Edinburgh.

CHAPTER 4

Cystic fibrosis: an overview

Berni Donaghy

Introduction

Cystic fibrosis (CF) is the most common, life-threatening, recessively inherited disease in the western world. It results from a gene mutation on the long arm of chromosome 7. It affects 1 in 2,500 Caucasians, which is approximately 1 live birth a day in the UK (Peckham and Conway, 2004) Approximately 1 in 25 people carry a CF gene mutation, which equates to around 2.3 million in the UK (http://www.cftrust.org.uk/). Over 1,000 mutations have been identified, although by far the most common in the Caucasian population (approximately 75%) is Delta F508 (http://www.cysticfibrosismedicine.com/).

Aetiology

The CF gene causes an abnormality in the production and function of a protein called the Cystic Fibrosis Transmembrane conductance Regulator (CFTR). Normally the CFTR regulates sodium, chloride and bicarbonate transport across cell membranes. CFTR is found in epithelial cells, which line the respiratory, gastrointestinal and reproductive tracts. Abnormal CFTR function leads to abnormal ion composition and relative dehydration of the surface liquid covering the epithelial cells. Widespread presence of CFTR helps to explain why CF is a multi-system condition (Peckham and Conway, 2004; Conway *et al.*, 2003). The two major organs affected are the lungs and the gastrointestinal tract (Conway *et al.*, 2003). The clinical severity of CF varies between patients with the same mutations in CFTR.

Pathology

Thick secretions are produced by the epithelial cells causing:

- Obstruction in the small airways, which leads to recurrent chest infections and bronchiectasis (see Chapter 3).
- Obstruction of the pancreatic duct, which causes destruction of the pancreas leading to pancreatic insufficiency.
- Sinus disease
- Failure of embryological development of the vas deferens.
- Bowel obstruction – meconium ileus and Distal Intestinal Obstruction Syndrome (DIOS).

Genetics

CF is an inherited disease; people who have cystic fibrosis are born with it. The abnormal gene is recessive; therefore two defective copies of the gene, one from each parent, are needed for a baby to be born with CF, and this means that both parents must be carriers of the defective CF gene (Box 4.1).

Box 4.1

If both parents are carriers, their child has:

- A one in four chance of being born with CF
- A two in four chance of being a carrier but not having CF
- A one in four chance of not having CF or being a carrier of the defective gene leading to infertility in male patients.

Source: http://www.cftrust.org.uk/

Screening

It is important that anyone who is classed as at high risk of having a baby with CF and is contemplating a pregnancy, or who has a newborn with CF, should be offered screening and early genetic advice.

Screening tests available (`http://www.cftrust.org.uk/`):

- Carrier testing – This can be carried out either by a blood sample or mouth brushing.
- Antenatal testing – via Chorionic Villus Sampling (CVS) or amniocentesis. This determines early in the pregnancy if the foetus has CF, and is usually offered to mothers recognised as being at high risk of having a child with CF (i.e. where both parents are carriers or there is a family history of CF).
- Neonatal testing – This is done on the heel prick test (Guthrie); however, not all regions are undertaking this at present.

Clinical presentation

Presentation depends on age. Typically cystic fibrosis presents in infancy, with a combination of failure to thrive, steatorrhoea and respiratory symptoms. At birth, 10–20% of patients present with meconium ileus, a blockage of the bowel caused by the sticky secretions (Peckham and Conway, 2004). However, CF can present and be diagnosed at any age. Adult males have been diagnosed at infertility clinics due to the absence of the vas deferens.

Confirmation of diagnosis

Diagnosis is made on clinical presentation together with a positive sweat test (Box 4.2).

All patients should be screened for known common CF gene mutations. This is known as genotyping. Identification of two CF gene mutations is absolute confirmation of the diagnosis (Hodson and Geddes, 2000). Neonatal screening for common CF mutations can be performed in a heel prick blood test, the Guthrie test, which all newborn will have performed soon after birth. Positive results can be further evaluated by examining the same blood spot for the presence of the common CF mutations (Ranieri *et al.*, 1994).

Complications

Cystic fibrosis is a multi-system disease with many complications.

Box 4.2 The sweat test (Hill, 1998)

The sweat test is the standard method of diagnosis, first described by Gibson and Cooke (1959) this comprises three components:

- Sweat induction
- Sweat collection
- Sweat analysis

Sweat chloride interpretation (mmol/l)

< 40	Normal – low probability of cystic fibrosis
40–60	Intermediate – suggestive but not diagnostic of cystic fibrosis
> 60	Elevated – supports the diagnosis of cystic fibrosis

Respiratory

The respiratory tract can be colonised with one or more bacteria (Box 4.3).

These are treated with individual or combinations of antibiotics depending on the bacteria grown and antibiotic sensitivities. Aggressive treatment with intravenous antibiotics to treat a respiratory exacerbation is advised. Antibiotics can also be given as a prophylactic measure in an attempt to prevent rather than treat the inevitable respiratory infections.

Box 4.3 Pathogens affecting the respiratory tract in CF

Bacteria: *Staphylococcus aureus*
Haemophilus influenzae
Streptococcus pneumonia
Pseudomonas aeruginosa
Burkhoderia cepacia
Mycobacterium tuberculosis
Klebsiella pneumoniae
Atypical mycobacterium
Stenotrophomonas maltophilia
Fungi: *Aspergillus*

In the lungs, poor clearance of thick secretions leads to recurrent infection, bronchial damage, bronchiectasis (see Chapter 3) and eventual death from respiratory failure. Box 4.4 illustrates the progression of the disease.

Box 4.4 Disease progression

Increased cough and sputum
Haemoptysis
Chest pain
Chronic dyspnoea
Finger clubbing
CXR: thickening of the bronchial walls
       Ill-defined nodular shadowing
Respiratory failure

Infection control

Owing to concerns about cross-infection between patients, the recommendations for CF care now include segregation according to microbiological status, not only in the clinic environment but also on the ward.

Gastro-intestinal

Gastro-oesophageal reflux and oesophagitis are common in CF (Hill, 1998). This may be due to lung disease, oesophageal dysmotility and delayed gastric emptying. Patients may be asymptomatic or present with anorexia, heartburn or reflux. Patients may be prescribed proton pump inhibitors (PPIs) or H_2 receptor agonists (H_2A) to alleviate symptoms.

Pancreatic complications

Approximately 90% of patients will have pancreatic insufficiency (PI) (Cystic Fibrosis Trust, 2002a). PI leads to malabsorption and maldigestion, causing impairment of pancreatic bicarbonate and chloride secretion and water flow into the duodenum. Without efficient pancreatic enzyme replacement, malabsorption leads to steatorrhoea, malnutrition and stunted growth, fat-soluble vitamin deficiency and delayed puberty. Patients are therefore routinely given enzyme replacement and Vitamins A, D and E.

Bowel obstruction syndrome

As a result of poor water flow, hyperconcentration of protein can occur and can lead to obstruction leading to a condition called Distal Intestinal Obstruction Syndrome (DIOS) (Cystic Fibrosis Trust, 2002a). Thick mucofaeculent material forms and obstructs the distal ileum, caecum and proximal colon (Conway *et al.*, 2003). It is reported to occur in 9–40% of patients (Conway *et al.*, 2003). The incidence appears to increase with age and is more common in adolescent and adult patients. Treatment, if the patient is tolerating oral intake, is a balanced intestinal lavage solution. In some cases surgical intervention is necessary.

Hepatic complications

Cirrhosis can occur arising from plugging of the small bile duct. Patients with liver disease are often asymptomatic. Splenomegaly, prominent abdominal veins, and a history of heamatemesis suggest portal hypertension. There is no proven therapy for liver disease. Medications such as ursodeoxycholic acid can improve biochemical dysfunction, but do not slow down progression.

The incidence of gallstones and other gall bladder disease is increased in CF (Peckham and Conway, 2004), and some patients may require surgery to correct biliary problems.

Reproductive

Almost all males with cystic fibrosis are infertile (Conway and Peckham, 2004) as a result of absence of the vas deferens, preventing transport of sperm from the epididymis to the prostate. However, sexual performance remains unaffected. The exact fertility status of women with cystic fibrosis is unclear. There is an increased chance of infertility due to increased thickness of cervical mucus (Conway and Peckham, 2004). Women are considered fertile and therefore require contraception; it is recommended that the contraceptive depot injection or a high-oestrogen oral contraceptive pill be prescribed.

Cystic fibrosis-related diabetes (CFRD)

Due to increasing survival in CF, pancreatic destruction resulting in insulin deficiency and diabetes mellitus is increasingly recognised. The prevalence of CFRD increases with age (Moran *et al.*, 1998; Lanng *et al.*, 1995) and occurs in up to 30% by age 25 (Peckham and Conway, 2004), with the average age of onset being 18–25 (Cystic Fibrosis Trust, 2003). It is slightly more common in females (Yung and Hodson, 1999; Rosenecker *et al.*, 1995). CFRD is distinct from types I and II diabetes but has features of each. It is associated with insulinopenia and insulin resistance (Hardin *et al.*, 2001) Ketoacidosis is unusual but can occur (Moran *et al.*, 1998). CFRD should be considered in patients with clinical decline and weight loss, and if undiagnosed can lead to decline in lung function. Some patients can have raised blood sugars only when unwell or when on corticosteroid therapy. Conflicts between dietary therapy of CF (see the section on nutrition below) and diabetes mellitus should be resolved in favour of the CF diet, i.e. they should not decrease their carbohydrate or fat intake. A CF specialist dietician normally sees all patients with CFRD on a regular basis. It is also advisable that patients are reviewed by a diabetologist at least annually.

CFRD is usually treated with insulin. Insulin therapy should be tailored to individual needs rather than diet tailored to insulin (Cystic Fibrosis Trust, 2004). It is recommended that patients over the age of 10 years should be screened for CFRD via an oral glucose tolerance test. This is the most accurate way of diagnosing diabetes mellitus (Etherington *et al.*, 2000; Verma *et al.*, 2002).

Nutrition

Adequate nutrition is vital for both quality of life and long-term survival. Evidence suggests a close relationship between nutritional status and lung function (Peckham and Conway, 2004; Hodson and Geddes, 2000; Cystic Fibrosis Trust, 2002a). Patients require a high-energy diet and should try to eat between 20–50% more kilocalories than the national recommendations for their age and sex (Cystic Fibrosis Trust, 2002a). Protein requirements are double the recommended adult intake with many patients. As lung function deteriorates nutritional support needs to become more aggressive, which may include overnight nasogastric or gastrostomy tube feeding. Enzyme replacement needs to be optimal at all times and it is extremely important that the CF specialist dietician reviews patients regularly.

Physiotherapy

Thick sputum causes recurrent infections and progressive lung damage. Physiotherapy aims to clear the sputum and minimise infection (Webber and Pryor, 1993) (Box 4.5). Patients tend to cough excessively to clear their chest, leading to fatigue and chest pain. Reduced ability to exercise and breathlessness are features of progressive lung disease, which physiotherapy can target (Bradley and Moran, 2002). CF patients can also suffer with joint pains, especially back problems, and females can suffer with stress incontinence due to weak pelvic floor muscles probably caused by excessive coughing (Orr *et al.*, 2001).

Box 4.5 The aims of physiotherapy in CF

■ To enable the patient to clear their chest as easily and effectively as possible with minimal coughing
■ To improve or maintain their exercise levels
■ To manage breathlessness
■ To minimise joint pains
■ To reduce or eliminate urinary incontinence

Physiotherapy techniques should be tailored to each patient's individual need, taking into consideration volume of sputum, wheeze and shortness of breath (Peebles, 1998). In CF the patient's preference for a particular physiotherapy technique is very important to promote concordance (Pryor, 1999). There are several techniques used to assist in chest clearance (Box 4.6). Timing of medication with chest physiotherapy is another important aspect; for example, taking nebulised DNase and bronchodilators before physiotherapy (Shak *et al.*, 1990), and nebulised antibiotics after chest physiotherapy.

Maintenance of cardiovascular fitness is important to keep limitation by breathlessness to a minimum (Peebles, 1998). Strength exercises maintain muscle strength and function, allowing them to use oxygen more effectively (O'Neill *et al.*, 1987). It is important that a specialist CF physiotherapist sees all patients and assesses them regularly (Cystic Fibrosis Trust, 2002b).

Box 4.6 Physiotherapy techniques

- Active cycle of breathing – A combination of gentle deep breathing exercise and huffing (forced expiration) to break up and move sputum
- Autogenic drainage – A complicated technique involving breathing at different lung volumes to clear sputum from all parts of the lungs.
- Flutter – A pipe shaped device that causes vibrating airflow when deep breathing through it, breaking up the sputum
- PEP – A device that produces a positive pressure when breathed through. This allows air to get behind sputum and move it.
- Acapella – Causes an oscillating, vibrating airflow, like the flutter, vibrations generated using a magnetic mechanism
- Postural drainage and percussion – especially with young children – Postural drainage involves lying in various positions using gravity to drain sputum. Percussion involves clapping the chest wall with a cupped hand. Dislodges sputum from the airway walls (usually combined with postural drainage)

Transition to adult care

Teenagers are usually transferred from paediatric to adult care between the ages of 16 and 18; this is an important milestone for both patient and family. It is imperative that there are strong relationships between the two centres to enable a smooth transition. Transition itself should be gradual, well-planned and coordinated, with full involvement of the patient and family. Interaction of parents and children with the adult team before transfer allows successful transition from paediatric to adult care.

Organisation of care

Unfortunately, specialist centres do not yet exist everywhere. The bulk of CF care should be undertaken by a specialist CF centre. If this is difficult due to lack of a local specialist multidisciplinary team, or the reluctance of the patient to travel long distances, patients are looked after via a shared care arrangement between a local hospital and major centre. However, patients should always be reviewed at least annually at a specialist CF centre. Box 4.7 highlights the optimum CF multidisciplinary team.

Box 4.7 The core CF team (Cystic Fibrosis Trust, 2002b)

Essential
Consultant Physician
Clinical Nurse Specialist
Specialist physiotherapist
Specialist dietician

Desirable
Specialist social worker
Psychologist
Pharmacist

Home Intravenous Antibiotic Therapy (HIVAT)

CF carries with it a huge burden of care, with treatment being daily and lifelong. Treatment concentrates on maximising lung function and nutritional status, with independence with treatment being encouraged from an early age.

Patients with CF experience repeated infective respiratory exacerbations, which are treated with intravenous antibiotics, normally given either via a long line or indwelling vascular access port. Some small studies have demonstrated that adequately supervised home intravenous antibiotic therapy (HIVAT) is a practical and effective alternative to hospital treatment for many patients with CF (Pond *et al.*, 1995; Bradley *et al.*, 1999; Esmond *et al.*, 2002; Riethmuller *et al.*, 2002). Other studies cite the advantages of HIVAT as: reduced risk of cross-infection, improved quality of life, and less time off school or work (Littlewood, 2000; Marco *et al.*, 2001). However, a larger study by Thornton *et al.* (2004) suggests that clinical outcomes (lung function, body weight) are better after a course of treatment as an inpatient than after home treatment.

Most patients (or carers) are taught how to constitute and administer their antibiotics aseptically. The first dose, and sometimes the second, should be administered in the hospital environment to observe for any anaphylactic reactions.

The cystic fibrosis nurse specialist (CFNS) is the central figure in the organisation of HIVAT (Cystic Fibrosis Trust, 2001). It is extremely important to ensure that the home environment is adequate before commencing such treatment and that there is support both for the patient and for the family.

Social issues

People with CF can find it difficult to gain employment. Employers have to be sympathetic to the needs of the CF sufferer, in respect of their daily routine, to fit in their numerous drugs and physiotherapy and the possibility of being hospitalised several times a year.

Many patients go to university, the choice of which is often being influenced by geographical location, accommodation needs and the availability of CF care local to the university.

Psychosocial impact of cystic fibrosis

The burden of living with a chronic and progressive disease can create enormous pressure, not only on the individual but also their family. Uncertainties about long-term prognosis can create feelings of isolation; it can also lead to rebellion and poor concordance with treatment. Adolescence in itself can take its toll on the healthy youngster, but to someone who is chronically ill this can have a devastating effect. Box 4.8 highlights a typical day in a CF patient's life.

Transplant

Transplant is considered when end-stage lung disease develops; around 90% of patients die from respiratory failure. To be considered for transplant patients must meet certain criteria (Box 4.9). Transplantation in itself is regarded as a palliative procedure, not a cure. The mean waiting time from acceptance onto a transplant programme to transplant itself is 12–24 months, while 50% of patients die while waiting for organs (Egan *et al.*, 2002).

End of life care

Even with optimal medical care, cystic fibrosis remains a life-limiting condition. The terminal stage can occur at any time from infancy to late adulthood. It

Box 4.8 A day in a CF patient's life

I am going to describe a typical day when I am working.

06:15 Get up and have nebulised DNase; takes approx. 10 mins (I have a small fridge upstairs to keep the DNase in to prevent me from having to use the stairs.
— Take 8 tablets, which must be taken on an empty stomach
— Shower and wash hair
07:00 Get dressed sitting on edge of the bed (I get my clothes out the night before so I don't need to bend into chest of drawers etc. when I am short of breath in the mornings
— Dry hair whilst nebulising ventolin
07:30 Autogenic drainage whilst nebulising saline (my husband usually brings me up a cup of tea and some Jammy Dodgers!!). Can take up to an hour, depending how tight my chest is.
08:00 Measure blood sugar and then take insulin
08:30 Nebulise antibiotic; takes approx. 20 mins
— Rinse in soapy water all nebuliser parts
09:00 Go downstairs and prepare and administer IV antibiotics
09:30–09:45 Prepare and eat breakfast. My husband gets everything out for me, so I just poach egg, cook bacon in the microwave, turn kettle on etc.
— Take tablets (13) and Creon (5)
10:00 Leave for work
14:45 Return from work
15:00 Prepare and administer IV antibiotics
15:30 Nebulise ventolin
— Go downstairs with sonic nebuliser and saline
— Do autogenic drainage (with a cup of tea and TV!!) for up to hour
— Nebulise antibiotic – 20 mins
— Rinse all nebuliser parts in soapy water
19:00 Evening meal, my husband usually prepares this meal on working days, as I am usually exhausted!!
21:00 Get tablets ready for tomorrow
— Have a bowl of cereal
21:30 Prepare and administer final IV dose
— Get all I need for morning dose before I go upstairs
22:00 BED!!

Box 4.9 Transplant criteria in CF (Egan et *al.*, 1998)

- FEV$_1$ 30% predicted
- Other important factors:
- Rate of decline in respiratory function
- Quality of life
- Increased need for intravenous therapy
- Poor weight profile

---

is usually recognised by increased severity and frequency of respiratory exacerbations, which can lead to oxygen dependence and declining lung function. Emphasis on care changes from aggressive treatment regimes to those focusing on symptom control. Patients deserve a pain-free and dignified death. Lung transplantation is an option in a few; however, the prospect of lung transplantation should never prevent good end of life care.

Conclusion

Fifty years ago, a baby born with CF might have survived for only a few months. Now, 75% of babies survive into adolescence and many well into adulthood (Elborn *et al.*, 2000). This is due to earlier diagnosis and improved treatments.

In the adult, CF is primarily a lung disorder, although it is imperative that all-round care is provided. Advances in the last 30 years have seen an advanced life expectancy and this is set to continue. In the next 10 years it is likely that the greater proportion of patients will be adults (Elborn *et al.*, 2000).

The future

With the isolation of the faulty gene, research in the past decade has centred on gene therapy to replace the defect. Research is still currently under way and the results awaited.

Acknowledgement

Cystic fibrosis multidisciplinary team, Glenfield Hospital, Leicester.

Useful address

Cystic Fibrosis Trust
11 London Road
Bromley
Kent
BR1 1BY
Email: enquiries@cftrust.org.uk
http://www.cftrust.org.uk/

Further reading

The following publications are all available from the Cystic Fibrosis Trust (http://www.cftrust.org.uk/):

Antibiotic Treatment for Cystic Fibrosis, 2nd edn
Burkholderia Cepacia
Clinical Guidelines for the Physiotherapy Management of Cystic Fibrosis
Management of Cystic Fibrosis Related Diabetes Mellitus
National Consensus Standards for the Nursing Management of Cystic Fibrosis
Nutritional Management of Cystic Fibrosis
Pseudomonas Aeruginosa Infection in People with Cystic Fibrosis
Standards for the Clinical Care of Children and Adults with Cystic Fibrosis in the UK

For articles and medicine database see http://www.cysticfibrosismedicine.com/

Bluebond-Langer, M., Lask, B. and Angst, D. B. (eds.) (2001) *Psychosocial Aspects of Cystic Fibrosis*. Arnold, London.
Hill, C. M. (1998) *Practical Guidelines for Cystic Fibrosis Care*. Churchill Livingstone, London.
Hodson, M. E. and Geddes, D. M. (2000) *Cystic Fibrosis*. Arnold, London.

References

Bradley, J. and Moran, F. (2002) Physical training for cystic fibrosis (Cochrane review). *The Cochrane Library*, Issue 4.

Bradley, J., Wallace, E., Elborn, J., Howard, J. L. and McCoy, M. P. (1999) An audit of the effect of intravenous antibiotic treatment on spirometric measures of pulmonary function in cystic fibrosis. *Irish Journal of Medical Science*, **168**, 25–8.

Conway, S. P., Littlewood, J. M., Brownlee, K. G., Peckham, D. G. and Members of the Leeds Regional Cystic Fibrosis Units (2003) *Cystic Fibrosis in Children and Adults. The Leeds Method of Management.* Revised edition No. 6, Forest Laboratories UK Limited.

Cystic Fibrosis Trust (2001) *National Consensus Standards For The Nursing Management of Cystic Fibrosis.* http://www.cftrust.org.uk/.

Cystic Fibrosis Trust (2002a) *Nutritional Management of Cystic Fibrosis.* http://www.cftrust.org.uk/.

Cystic Fibrosis Trust (2002b) *Clinical Guidelines for the Physiotherapy Management of Cystic Fibrosis.* http://www.cftrust.org.uk/.

Cystic Fibrosis Trust (2004) *Management of Cystic Fibrosis Related Diabetes Mellitus.* http://www.cftrust.org.uk/.

Egan, T. M., Detterbeck, S. C., Mill, M. R., Gott, K. K., Rea, J. B., McSweeney, J., Aris, R. M. and Paradowski, L. J. (1998) Lung transplantation for cystic fibrosis: effective and durable therapy in a high-risk group. *Annals of Thoracic Surgery*, **66**, 337–46.

Egan, T. M., Detterbeck, S. C., Mill, M. R., Bleiweis, M. A., Aris, R., Paradowski, L., Retsch-Bogart, G., Mueller, B. S., Neuringer, I. and Rivera, M. P. (2002) Long term results of lung transplantation for cystic fibrosis. *European Journal of Cardiothoracic Surgery*, **22**, 602–9.

Elborn, J. S., Shale, D. J. and Britton, J. R. (2000) Cystic fibrosis: current survival and population estimates to year 2000. *Thorax*, **46**, 881–5.

Esmond, G., Butler, M., McCormack, A. and Empey, D. (2002) Comparison of hospital and home intravenous antibiotic therapy in adults with cystic fibrosis. Journal of Cystic Fibrosis, **1** (suppl. 1), 326.

Etherington, C., Morton, A., White, H., Peckham, D. and Conway, S. P. (2000). Screening for CFRD. *Abstract book, XIIIth International Cystic Fibrosis Conference.* Abs. 134.

Gibson, L. E. and Cooke, R. E. (1959) In: *Practical Guidelines for Cystic Fibrosis Care* (1998; ed. C. M. Hill), Chapter 21. Churchill Livingstone, London.

Hardin, D. S., LeBlanc, A., Lukenbaugh, S. and Seilheimer, D. K. (2001) Mechanisms of insulin resistance in cystic fibrosis. *American Journal of Physiology, Endocrinology and Metabolism*, **281**, 1022–8.

Hill, C. M. (ed.) (1998) *Practical Guidelines for Cystic Fibrosis Care.* Churchill Livingstone, London.

Hodson, M. E. and Geddes, D. M. (2000) *Cystic Fibrosis.* Arnold, London.

Lanng, S., Hansen, A., Thorsteinsson, B., Nerup, J. and Koch, C. (1995) Glucose tolerance in patients with cystic fibrosis: five year prospective study. *British Medical Journal*, **311**, 655–9.

Littlewood, J. M. (2000) Good care for people with cystic fibrosis. *Paediatric Respiratory Reviews*, **1**, 179–89.

Moran, A., Doherty, L., Wang, X. and Thomas, W. (1998) Abnormal glucose metabolism in cystic fibrosis. Journal of Pediatrics, **133**, 10–17.

Marco, T., Asensio, O., Bosque, M., De Gracia, J. and Serra, C. (2001) Home intravenous antibiotics for cystic fibrosis (Cochrane review). *The Cochrane Library*, Issue 1.

O'Neil, P., Dodd, M. and Phillips, B. (1987) Regular exercise and reduction of breathlessness in patients with cystic fibrosis. *British Journal of Diseases of the Chest*, **81**, 62–9.

Orr, A., McKean, R. J., Webb, A. K. and Dodd, M. E. (2001) Questionnaire survey of urinary incontinence in women with cystic fibrosis. British Medical Journal, **322**, 1521.

Peckham, D. and Conway S. (2004) Cystic fibrosis. *Medicine*, **32**(1), 124–8.

Peebles A. (1998) Physiotherapy. In: *Practical Guidelines for Cystic Fibrosis Care* (ed. C. M. Hill), Chapter 5. Churchill Livingstone, London.

Pond, M., Newport, M., Joanes, D. and Conway, S. P. (1995) Home versus hospital intravenous antibiotic therapy in the treatment of young adults with cystic fibrosis. *European Respiratory Journal*, **7**, 1640–4.

Pryor, J. A. (1999) Physiotherapy for airway clearance in adults. *European Respiratory Journal*, **14**, 1418–24.

Ranieri, E., Lewis, B. D. and Gerace, R. I. (1994) Neonatal screening for cystic fibrosis using immunoreactive trypinogen and direct gene analysis: four years experience. *British Medical Journal*, **308**, 1469–72.

Riethmuller, J., Busch, A., Damm, V., Ziebach, R. and Stern, M. (2002) Home and hospital antibiotic treatment prove similarly effective in cystic fibrosis. *Infection*, **30**, 387–91.

Rosenecker, J., Eichler, I., Kuhn, L., Harms, H. K. and von der Hardt, H. (1995) Genetic determination of diabetes mellitus in patients with cystic fibrosis. Journal of Pediatrics, **127**, 441–3.

Shak, S., Capon, D. J., Hellmiss, R., Marsters, S. A. and Baker, C. L. Recombinant human DNase I reduces viscosity of cystic fibrosis sputum. *Proceedings of the National Academy of Sciences USA*, **87**, 9188–92.

Thornton, J., Elliot, R., Tully, M. P. and Dodd, M. (2004) Long-term clinical outcome of home and hospital intravenous antibiotic treatment in adults with cystic fibrosis. *Thorax*, **59**, 242–6.

Verma, A., Claridge, A., Havelock, T., Biesty, J., McMenna, D. and Webb, A. K. Re-audit of the screening protocol for cystic fibrosis related diabetes (CFRD) in an adult centre. *Thorax*, **57**(suppl. 11), iii20.

Webber, B. A. and Pryor, J. A. (1993) *Physiotherapy for Respiratory and Cardiac Problems*. Churchill Livingstone, London.

Yunng, B. and Hodson, M. E. (1999) Diabetes in cystic fibrosis. *Journal of the Royal Society of Medicine*, **92**(suppl. 37), 35–40.

CHAPTER 5

Chronic obstructive pulmonary disease

Sue Burton

Aetiology/epidemiology

About 30 million working days are lost and 30,000 people die each year in the UK alone from chronic obstructive pulmonary disease (COPD) (Halpin, 2001). Globally there are 3 million deaths per year from COPD (Bourke, 2003). COPD is the only common cause of death that is still rising dramatically in the UK, and in the next few years it is thought that it will become the third most common cause of all deaths (World Health Organization, 2006).

It is estimated that 15% of men and 5% of women in the UK have COPD, and this is a becoming a major health burden, stretching our health care services and resources (Halpin, 2001). Currently 25% of all hospital admissions are due to respiratory disease and half of these are due to COPD. This results in the use of over one million bed days per year (British Thoracic Society, 2006).

What is it?

COPD is an umbrella term used to describe any respiratory condition causing longstanding fixed airflow obstruction which is non- or only partially reversible with bronchodilator therapy (National Collaborating Centre for Chronic Conditions, 2004). This spectrum of diseases includes chronic bronchitis and emphysema, although each of these diseases has a different pathological process (Bourke, 2003).

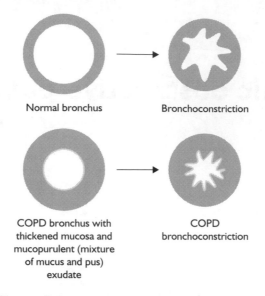

Normal bronchus   Bronchoconstriction

COPD bronchus with   COPD
thickened mucosa and   bronchoconstriction
mucopurulent (mixture
of mucus and pus)
exudate

Figure 5.1 Effects of COPD on the airways.

Patients with COPD have an exaggerated inflammatory response in the airways and parenchyma of the lung secondary to the years of inhaling cigarette smoke or noxious materials. These oxidative irritants cause damage to the respiratory epithelium, resulting in an influx of macrophages to the area of damage. The damage also causes neutrophils to be released from the blood stream. These neutrophils and macrophages release proteases and elastases, which cause a breakdown of connective tissue. In the long term the inflammation and then repair is associated with proteolysis, fibrosis and remodelling of the airways and lung parenchyma. Inflammation of the central airways, resulting in chronic mucus production and a chronic cough, is termed bronchitis, whereas the processes of destruction and repair in the respiratory bronchioles and alveoli cause emphysema. Many patients with COPD have a degree of both of these underlying pathological processes.

Furthermore, destruction of the capillary bed surrounding the alveoli and inflammation of pulmonary artery vessels cause pulmonary artery hypertension and, in turn, right-sided heart failure, cor pulmonale.

What causes it?

COPD is mainly associated with cigarette smoking, with around 90% of all cases having a substantial smoking history of more than twenty pack years (Bellamy and Booker, 2003)

To calculate the pack years for a person who smokes 30 cigarettes a day for 40 years, use the formula

$$A \times B = \text{pack years}$$

where

$$A = \text{packs per day} = \text{number of cigarettes per day}/20$$
$$B = \text{years of smoking}$$

Thus in our example:

$$A = 30/20 = 1.5$$
$$B = 40$$
$$\text{So pack years} = 1.5 \times 40 = 60$$

Tobacco use in the UK is a major health burden. Currently there are about 10 million adult cigarette smokers and 1 million pipe and cigar smokers (ASH, 2006). Although cigarette smoking is not the only cause of COPD, it is a major contributor, with 90% of deaths from COPD attributable to smoking (Hansel and Barnes, 2004). Despite these figures, only 15% of smokers actually develop COPD, suggesting that other causes may be involved, such as environmental factors (including coal dust and pollution), factors in early childhood, and genetic factors. Genetic factors are at present poorly defined except in the case of deficiency of anti-protease enzymes (Alpha 1 antitrypsin).

Clinical picture

The main clinical symptoms are breathlessness or dyspnoea, cough and sputum production, but a substantial degree of lung damage can take place before clinical symptoms become obvious. Indeed, most patients with COPD will have experienced a 50% decrease in FEV_1 before they present with their symptoms (Bellamy and Booker, 2002).

Breathlessness

Breathlessness occurs in patients with COPD due to the increased work of breathing caused by narrowing of the airways. This can affect distribution of

Table 5.1 MRC scale (adapted from Fletcher *et al.*, 1959).

Grade	Degree of breathlessness related to activities
1	Not troubled by breathlessness except on strenuous exercise
2	Short of breath when hurrying or walking up a slight hill
3	Walks slower than contemporaries on level ground because of breathlessness, or has to stop for breath when walking at own pace
4	Stops for breath after walking about 100 m or after a few minutes on level ground
5	Too breathless to leave the house, or breathless when dressing or undressing

air within the lungs, altering ventilation-to-perfusion matching, which in turn reduces gas exchange.

Breathlessness is often described as the most important and common symptom, but unfortunately it correlates poorly with physiological measurement. It is important to remember that patients with the most severe measured lung function are not necessarily the ones who report the greatest experience of breathlessness (Mahler *et al.*, 1984). Breathlessness is a subjective experience and can be influenced by more than just physical effects. Psychological effects have a large impact upon a patient's breathlessness and it is often difficult to differentiate the physical components of breathlessness from the social, psychological and spiritual components (Ahmedzai, 2004). This reinforces the importance of assessing, treating and planning patient care with a holistic approach. One method of ascertaining a patient's breathlessness is to use a tool such as the MRC scale that can assess the patients own perceived disability related to their breathlessness (Table 5.1).

Cough

Patients with COPD may present with a chronic productive cough, although this can be ignored by the patient and often attributed to being a 'smoker's cough'. The cough is frequently worse in the winter months and the patient may report a history of 'winter bronchitis' lasting many years.

The cough need not necessarily be always productive and many patients may present with a dry cough.

Cough is caused by an irritation of the airway nerves due to a release of compounds from inflammatory cells or by the presence of increased sputum production due to increased mucus secretion.

Table 5.2 Other symptoms of COPD.

- Hypoxia – decreased levels of PaO_2
- Fatigue – due to increased work of breathing
- Depression – due to exercise limitation, frustration and social isolation
- Chest tightness – often after exertion
- Chest pains – may be due to ischaemic heart disease or muscle strain
- Oedema – can indicate right-sided heart failure
- Wheeze – often found in severe COPD or during exacerbations caused by the sound generated by turbulent airflow through the airways due to the increased presence of sputum
- Weight loss and anorexia – often in advanced disease due to the increased work of breathing and nutritional depletion
- Muscle weakness – often due to poor conditioning. May be attributed to circulating cytokines

Sputum

Sputum production may be purulent, particularly during exacerbations, and this is often difficult to assess if patients do not monitor this. Patients should be advised to observe sputum for colour, consistency and volume, as any variation from their normal may be the first indication of an exacerbation.

Table 5.2 lists some other symptoms of COPD.

Exacerbations

COPD is not a stable disease and patients have symptoms and functional ability that vary from day to day (Morgan, 2003). Periods of worsening are termed 'exacerbations' and these occur on average between one and four times a year for each patient (Wedzicha, 2002). This can result in frequent hospital admissions. As the disease becomes more severe, patients experience more frequent exacerbations with less time between each one, indicating a more palliative phase of their illness.

Exacerbations may be caused by bacterial or viral infections, but often there is no apparent cause. It is suggested that continued cigarette smoking or an increase in air pollution may contribute.

Exacerbations are often dealt with in the community as there are more services available to treat patients at home. These are services often managed by nurses and physiotherapists, and such services have been proven to be a cost-effective, safe way of treating a patient at home (Burton, 2004).

Physical examination

Patents with COPD are often classified as either 'Pink Puffers' or 'Blue Bloaters'; however, many patients have a mixed picture. These labels are old terms but are still frequently used to describe patients with COPD (Table 5.3).

Chest auscultation may demonstrate reduced breath sounds, crepitations early in inspiration and a wheeze which may be present during inspiration and expiration. Many patients with symptomatic COPD have a prolonged expiratory time of more than 4 seconds. Patients may also have ankle oedema or an increased JVP, which indicates pulmonary artery hypertension or cor pulmonale.

Table 5.3 Clinical features of chronic bronchitis and emphysema.

Chronic bronchitis (Blue Bloater)	Emphysema (Pink Puffer)
■ Persistent cough productive of sputum	■ No cough or a dry cough
■ Overweight	■ Thin or cachetic
■ Can get cor pulmonale	■ Can get cor pulmonale
■ Obstruction on exhalation	■ Difficulty exhaling
■ Blue complexion (cyanosis)	■ Pink complexion (no cyanosis)
■ Recurrent infections	■ Frequent exacerbations but no infection
■ Polycythemia	■ No polycythemia

Investigations

A diagnosis of COPD should be made on clinical features and symptoms along with the evidence of airflow obstruction. This can be obtained by simple spirometry (Chapter 11).

The British Thoracic Society recommends that GPs should consider screening every patient at risk from COPD, especially smokers over the age of 35, with spirometry (British Thoracic Society, 2005).

Table 5.4 Classification of COPD (NCCCC, 2004).

- In MILD disease there are few symptoms, with a history of a morning cough, recurrent respiratory infections and shortness of breath on vigorous exercise; FEV_1 is 50–80% of predicted normal.

- In MODERATE disease, a wide range of symptoms present themselves, such as cough, production of sputum, acute worsening of symptoms of infection, wheeze and over-inflation of the lungs; and FEV_1 is 30–50% of predicted normal.

- In SEVERE disease there is breathlessness on minimal exertion, cough, wheeze, loss of weight, central cyanosis, peripheral oedema, pulmonary hypertension and over-inflation of the lungs; FEV_1 is less than 30% predicted normal.

COPD is categorised into three main classes, depending on the severity of the disease according to spirometry (Table 5.4).

Further tests and investigations can be performed, including chest X-ray, which in COPD should demonstrate large hyper-inflated lungs with flattened diaphragms.

High-resolution computerised tomography (CT) scans can demonstrate the pattern of emphysema and distribution throughout the lung fields. Further lung function tests can demonstrate reductions in transfer factor for carbon dioxide and transfer coefficient in physiological tests.

Arterial blood gases commonly reveal hypoxaemia (low oxygen levels) and hypercapnia (high carbon dioxide levels) (Chapter 14).

Complications of COPD

Cor pulmonale

Right-sided heart failure is caused by an enlargement of the right ventricle secondary to primary pulmonary disease. The right side of the heart has to work harder to maintain the circulation because of the increased pulmonary resistance caused by narrowing of the pulmonary capillaries. Over time this leads to hypertrophy and then failure of the right ventricle, causing peripheral oedema as fluid is pushed out of the capillaries into the tissues.

In the early stages, cor pulmonale usually presents as ankle oedema.

As the condition worsens, the oedema can spread up the legs and lower trunk. The presence of peripheral oedema in COPD is indicative of a poor prognosis.

Pneumothorax

This is the presence of air in the pleural cavity. In COPD this may occur spontaneously, as a specific result of emphysema. In advanced emphysema the damaged alveoli can form bullae, and if a bulla ruptures into the pleural cavity the result is total deflation of the affected lung.

Polycythaemia

When there are chronically low levels of oxygen in the circulation, this can result in an increase in the number of red blood cells. This increases the oxygen-carrying capacity of the blood, but also increases its viscosity and may make the patient more liable to pulmonary embolism. The polycythaemia may be managed by removing several units of blood, known as venesection.

Management

Nursing

Nursing interventions include psychological support and the supportive care of educating the patient and their family in ways of managing the disease. The most important nursing intervention is smoking cessation as this can have a large benefit for the patient's prognosis (see Chapter 15). Nurses also play a part in education of the patient and their family with medications. Advice about medications and lifestyle changes can have a large impact upon quality of life and breathlessness. Simple measures, such as advising patients about energy conservation techniques, when to ask for help and benefits they may be entitled to, may result in a large gain for the patient and their carers.

Nutrition

Patients who have COPD may be malnourished due to their increased work of breathing and can have nutritional depletion as they may feel too breathless to eat or chew. Advice on selection of foods, eating small regular meals or making use of oxygen during meals may help with nutritional problems and a Body Mass Index (BMI) should always be calculated. If the BMI is abnormal (high or low), or changing over time, the patient should be referred for dietetic advice. If the BMI is low, patients should also be given nutritional supplements to increase their total calorific intake, and be encouraged to take exercise to augment the effects of nutritional supplementation.

Physiotherapy

As well as being instructed on the use of exercise, patients can be taught chest clearance techniques to help aid expectoration. Help with posture and range of movement can be beneficial, as some areas of the cervical and thoracic spine and the shoulders are particularly vulnerable to stiffness due to breathlessness, and the overuse of accessory muscles can affect posture. These areas are assessed and exercises given where necessary to minimise loss of lung capacity. Physiotherapy can also help with breathing control and positioning.

Occupational therapy (OT)

Occupational therapy input for patients with COPD includes management of activities of daily living (ADLs), energy conservation and pacing. Patients can be assessed for energy expenditure and equipment to assist with ADLs as required. OTs can also provide relaxation and stress management techniques for patients that require help with this.

Medical

COPD is a progressive incurable disease and any treatment given is palliative rather than curative, with an intention to relive dyspnoea and improve functional status and quality of life. Optimal medical management involves a number of supportive treatments with primary goals of (Hansel and Barnes, 2004):

- Symptom relief
- Maintenance of functional activity level
- Prevention of complications
- Slowing the natural progression of the disease

Table 5.5 Criteria for referral for consideration for surgery (NCCCC, 2004).

- FEV_1 more than 20% predicted
- $PaCO_2$ less than 7.3 kPa
- Upper lobe predominant emphysema
- TLCO more than 20% predicted

The main pharmacological interventions include bronchodilators, mucolytics, corticosteroids and antibiotics for infections, vaccines and long-term supplemental oxygen for hypoxic patients (Jeffries and Turley, 1999).

Surgical options for patients with COPD are limited. Patients who have a single large bulla on a CT scan and an FEV_1 less than 50% predicted should be referred for consideration of bullectomy, and patients with severe COPD who remain breathless with marked restrictions of their activities of daily living despite maximal medical therapy should be referred for consideration of lung volume reduction surgery if they meet the correct criteria (Table 5.5).

Prognosis/outcome

COPD is a progressive disease with no known cure although there are methods to try and delay this deterioration.

Degree of airway obstruction can possibly be related to survival rates. The most severe cases, with an FEV_1 of less than 20% predicted, have the worst survival rates (Anthonisen *et al.*, 1986; Senoir and Anthonisen, 1998). These survival rates are accelerated if a patient has a faster rate of decline of FEV_1.

Stopping smoking is the single most important factor that a patient can address to help try to slow the progress of the disease. A key feature for improving a patient's functional capability is pulmonary rehabilitation (Chapter 12).

Patients with end stage COPD should be referred to specialist palliative care teams to assist with end of life issues and support.

Psychology/education

All patients should receive smoking cessation advice at every opportunity (see Chapter 15). They should also receive information about medication and its uses, and in the long term this may improve concordance. Education about the correct usage of inhaler devices can help patients to get maximum benefit from their medications.

Education about lifestyle changes and breathlessness can help patients to cope with their disease, and even simple advice about taking inhalers or nebulisers before exertion or how to manage ADLs can make a large impact on the patient's day-to-day tasks and improve their quality of life.

Case study

Mr Brown is a 68-year-old retired driver with a 75 pack year smoking history. His disease severity level upon admission to hospital was severe. He was on 2 L/min of oxygen for 24 hours a day. He admits to still smoking 'on occasion, when I am under stress'. Mr Brown has been housebound for two years because of his need for oxygen (via a concentrator) and fear of being too far from his nebuliser. He didn't have a Salbutamol inhaler in the house that was in date.

The COPD nurses worked with Mr Brown to address his needs. After communication with his doctor, he was given a prescription for a new Salbutamol and ipratropium inhaler with a spacer device. The nurse provided him with detailed instruction on the proper use of a spacer device and he found that with the correct technique he could achieve nearly the same effect he was getting in his nebuliser. The nurse talked through with Mr Brown that if he was still experiencing symptoms a long-acting bronchodilator would be added to his treatment and that a combination inhaler of a long acting bronchodilator and inhaled corticosteroid would be considered for continuing symptoms or if he was experiencing exacerbations. He was also provided with a portable oxygen cylinder to leave the house. He was referred to the OT for anxiety management and energy conservation techniques and received help from the physiotherapists about breathing control.

The nurses educated him on the vital importance of exercise and complete smoking cessation in slowing the progression of COPD, and he was enrolled upon the local pulmonary rehabilitation program. During the past year, his exercise tolerance has increased from 5-minute walks three times a week to 15–20 minute walks four or five times a week. He feels comfortable taking short trips outside the home with his wife and grandchild for the first time in years. The patient has reiterated that his change in lifestyle has led to an increase in quality of life. His oxygen needs at rest have decreased and he mainly uses it during activity and sleep. He also feels prepared to commit to complete smoking cessation at this time.

Activities

1. Find a patient with COPD and discuss with them their main symptoms and how this limits them in day to day activities. Can you think of any ways to help them overcome these problems
2. Try and collect as many different placebo inhaler devices as you can (drugs reps often have a stock of these) and then find a patient and ask them to demonstrate their inhaler technique. Do they use the device correctly? If not why not? Have they ever received proper instructions before?
3. Find out about local palliative care services and see what they offer for patient with non-malignant disease.

Key points

- COPD is a common condition, having a major impact on patients, carers and healthcare resources.
- COPD is a terminal disease and kills 3 million people each year.
- Because mild COPD is largely symptomatic, significant and irreversible damage is often already present at the time of diagnosis.
- The main cause of COPD is cigarette smoke.
- Smoking cessation is the only treatment that has been shown to alter disease progression. For the continuing smoker the prognosis is one of progressive decline into respiratory failure.
- The main symptoms are cough and breathlessness.
- Treatment is essentially palliative to ensure maximum functional capacity within the limitations of the disease.
- Bronchodilators are the cornerstone of the pharmaceutical management of COPD, although steroids may have a part to play in a minority of patients.
- Exercise, education and support are equally important in overall management. They confer significant benefits when they are part of an integrated pulmonary rehabilitation programme.
- Long-term oxygen therapy relieves symptoms and reduces mortality when used in patients with severe respiratory impairment.

References

Ahmedzai, S. (1999) Palliation of respiratory symptoms. In *Oxford Textbook of Palliative Medicine*, 2nd edn (eds. D. Doyle, G. Hanke and N. MacDonald). Oxford University Press, New York.

Anthonisen, N. R., Wright, E. C. and Hodgkin, J. E. (1986) Prognosis in chronic obstructive pulmonary disease. *American Review of Respiratory Disease*, **133**(1), 14–20.

ASH (2006) Factsheet no. 1: *Smoking statistics: Who smokes and how much.* http://www.ash.org.uk/html/factsheets/html/fact01.html

Bellamy, D. and Booker, R. (2002) *Chronic Obstructive Pulmonary Disease in Primary Care*, 2nd edn. Class Health, London.

Bourke, S. J. (2003) *Respiratory Medicine*, 6th edn. Blackwell, Oxford.

British Thoracic Society (2005) *Spirometry in Practice – A Practical Guide*, 2nd edn. British Thoracic Society COPD Consortium, London.

Burton, S. L. (2004) Early discharge of people with chronic obstructive pulmonary disease. *Nursing Times*, **100**(6), 65.

Fletcher, C. M., Elmes, P. C., Fairbairn, M. B. and Wood, C. H. (1959) The significance of respiratory symptoms and the diagnosis of chronic bronchitis in a working population. *British Medical Journal*, **2**, 257–66.

Halpin, D. M. G. (2001) *COPD*. Harcourt.

Hansel, T. T. and Barnes, P. J. (2004) *An Atlas of Chronic Obstructive Pulmonary Disease*. Parthenon Publishing, London.

Jeffries, A. and Turley, A. (1999) *Mosby's Crash Course Respiratory System*. Mosby, Edinburgh.

Mahler, D., Weinberg, D., Wells, C. and Feinstein, A. R. (1984) The measurement of dyspnoea. Contents, interobserver agreement, and physiologic correlates of two new clinical indexes. *Chest*, **85**(6), 751–8.

Morgan, M. D. L. (2003) Preventing hospital admissions for COPD: role of physical activity. *Thorax*, **58**, 95–6.

National Collaborating Centre for Chronic Conditions (2004) Chronic obstructive pulmonary disease; national clinical guidelines for management of chronic obstructive pulmonary disease in adults in primary and secondary care. *Thorax*, **54**(suppl. 1), 1–232.

Senior, R. M. and Anthonisen, N. R. (1998) Chronic obstructive pulmonary disease. *American Journal of Respiratory Critical Care Medicine*, **157**(4), S139–47.

Wedzicha, J. A. (2002) Exacerbations, etiology and pathophysiologic mechanisms. *Chest*, **121**(5), S136–41.

World Health Organization (WHO) (2006) *COPD: Burden.* http://www.who.int/respiratory/copd/burden/en/index.html

Suggested further reading

British Thoracic Society (1997) Guidelines for the management of chronic obstructive pulmonary disease. *Thorax*, **52**, Supplement 5.

British Thoracic Society (2006) *The Burden of Lung Disease*, 2nd edn. British Thoracic Society. http://www.brit-thoracic.org.uk/c2/uploads/finalproof.pdf

Coakley, A. L. (2001a) Pulmonary disease and smoking: a case for health promotion. *British Journal of Nursing*, **10**(1), 20–4.

Coakley, A. L. (2001b) Helping patients to master correct inhaler techniques: nursing role. *British Journal of Nursing*, **10**(7), 424–32.

Esmond, G. (1998) Nebuliser therapy. *Professional Nurse*, **14**(1), 39–43.

Gravil, J. H., Al-Rowans, O. A., Cotton, M. M., Flanigan, U., Irwin, A. and Stevenson, R. D. (1998) Home treatment of exacerbations of Chronic Obstructive Pulmonary Disease by an acute respiratory assessment service. *Lancet*, **351**(June), 1853–5.

Guthrie, S. J., Hill, K. M. and Muers, M. F. (2001) Living with severe COPD. A qualitative exploration of the experience of patients in Leeds. *Respiratory Medicine*, **95**, 196–204.

Lynn, J., Ely, E. W., Zhong, Z., McNiff, K. L., Dawson, N. V., Connors, A., Desbiens, N. A., Claessens, M. and McCarthy, E. P. (2000) Living and dying with chronic obstructive pulmonary disease. *Journal of the American Geriatric Society*, **48**(5), S910–S1000.

McAllister, J. (2002a) Chronic obstructive pulmonary disease: foundation epidemiology and disease process, anatomy and physiology, signs and symptoms. *Nursing Times* **98**(35), 41–4.

McAllister, J. (2002b) Chronic obstructive pulmonary disease: diagnosis and assessment, investigations and treatments, *Nursing Times*, **98**(36), 27–30.

McAllister, J. (2002c) Chronic obstructive pulmonary disease: nursing care and implications for nursing. *Nursing Times*, **98**(37), 43–5.

Seemungal, T. A., Donaldson, G. C., Paul, E. A., Bestall, J. C., Jeffries, D. J. and Wedzicha, J. A. (1998) Effect of exacerbation on quality of life in patients with chronic obstructive pulmonary disease. *American Journal of Respiratory Critical Care Medicine*, **157**, 1418–22.

Skwarska, E., Cohen, G., Skwarski, K. M., Lamb, C., Bushell, D., Parekt, S. and MacNee, W. (2000) Randomised controlled trial of supported discharge in patients with exacerbations of chronic obstructive pulmonary disease. *Thorax*, **55**, 907–12.

CHAPTER 6

Lung cancer

Liz Darlison

Introduction

In 2001, more than 270,000 new cases of cancer were registered in the UK. There are over 200 different types of cancer and it is the cause of 26% of all deaths in the UK (Cancer Research UK, 2005).

One in three people will be diagnosed with cancer during their lifetime. However, it is a disease that affects mainly older people, with 64% of cases occurring in those aged 65 and over. As the average life expectancy in the UK has almost doubled since the mid-nineteenth century the population at risk of cancer has grown.

Lung cancer is the second most commonly diagnosed cancer in the UK. In 2001 there were 37,450 new cases, accounting for 14% of all cancers diagnosed (Cancer Research UK, 2005).

Whilst the incidence of lung cancer is less than that for breast cancer, lung cancer deaths account for more than a fifth of all cancer deaths. In 2002 this amounted to 33,600 lung cancer deaths, or 22% of all cancer deaths (Cancer Research UK, 2004). On average, 92 people die every day from lung cancer in the UK (Cancer Research UK, 2005).

Causes

Cigarette smoking has been identified as the single most important cause of preventable disease and premature death in the UK. Overall, a third of all cancer deaths are linked to smoking.

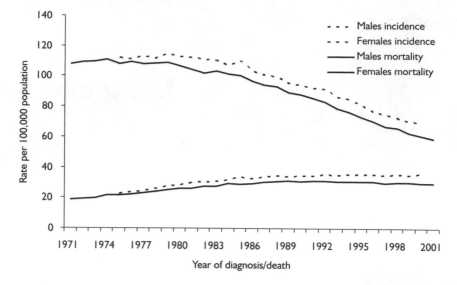

Figure 6.1 Age standardised (European) incidence and mortality per 100,000 population, lung cancer, by sex, Great Britain, 1971–2002 (`http://www.can-cerresearchuk.org/`).

Trends in smoking habits directly correlate to incidence and mortality in lung cancer. Male lung cancer rates have continued to decrease since the early 1970s (Figure 6.1) and during this time the prevalence of men smoking has dropped from 51% to 26% (Cancer Research UK, 2004). Female lung cancer rates increased until the early 1990s. They have now reached a plateau and stayed reasonably stable (Figure 6.1). This trend is directly attributed to the increase in females who have become addicted to smoking. Cancer Research UK (2004) reports that girls continue to be more likely to smoke than boys, with 11% of girls aged 11–15 years smoking compared to 8% of boys.

Not only are females more likely to smoke, but Patel *et al.* (2004) warns that lung cancer appears to be a different disease in women than men. Patel *et al.* claim that female smokers are more at risk of developing adenocarcinoma of the lung due to the presence of a novel oestrogen receptor that has been identified in lung tumours, which may be stimulated by the naturally occurring hormone. In addition, female smokers are known to have increased levels of a gene called *CYP1A1* which makes cigarette smoke chemicals harmful to cells, and they also have a reduced ability to repair DNA than men.

The smoking habits of women and Patel *et al.*'s findings should perhaps be considered by nurses when evaluating or screening patients who smoke and when planning smoking cessation programmes.

It must be remembered, however, that lung cancer is not exclusive to smokers. If it is accepted, as reported by Brogden (1998), that 10% of lung cancer is not due to smoking, in 2002 there were 3,500 lung cancer deaths that were not related to smoking. Non-smoking-related lung cancer is therefore a significant disease, responsible for more deaths than malignant melanoma or cancer of the testicle, cervix, head and neck, or liver.

Signs and symptoms

Lung cancer can grow silently for years without causing any ill effects. Symptoms are often subtle and easily attributed to a cold or bronchitis, particularly when patients have pre-existing chronic obstructive pulmonary disease or are a smoker (Box 6.1). The link between smoking and lung cancer means there is a stigma attached to the disease and this can lead patients to deny symptoms for some time before seeking help. Patients should be encouraged to observe for new symptoms but also any small, subtle change in chronic symptoms.

Early detection will continue to depend on increasing the public's awareness of the signs and symptoms of lung cancer and encouraging patients to seek help as soon as possible. There is no recognised method suitable for mass screening for lung cancer. Further trials are required before any screening methods are introduced into clinical practice.

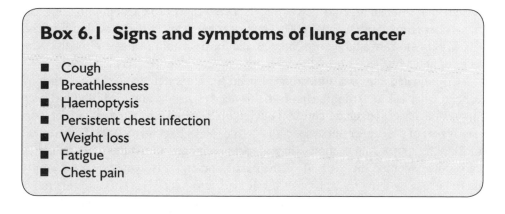

Box 6.1 Signs and symptoms of lung cancer

- Cough
- Breathlessness
- Haemoptysis
- Persistent chest infection
- Weight loss
- Fatigue
- Chest pain

Referral to hospital

Patients with lung cancer, at the time of diagnosis, present to hospital in a number of different ways (Box 6.2).

Melling *et al.* (2002) in a random sample of 400 patients with lung cancer discovered that different referral routes into hospital are associated with different rates of investigation, treatment and management of patients. The rec-

Box 6.2 Routes for hospital referral

- GP (two-week wait)
- Accident and emergency
- Medical Admissions Unit
- Routine admission (abnormal chest X-ray)
- Other specialist outpatient department clinic

ommendations are that all patients with suspected lung cancer, regardless of their age or other health problems, should be seen by a respiratory physician. Fergusson *et al.* (2003) studied 3855 lung cancer patients and concluded that the 75% that were seen by a respiratory physician were more likely to have a histological confirmed diagnosis and to have had active treatment with surgery, chemotherapy or radiotherapy. More were alive at one year and benefits were found to have remained three years after diagnosis.

Guidelines from the British Thoracic Society (BTS) (1998) and the National Health Service (NHS) Executive (1998) also recommend that all patients with lung cancer receive prompt care. The NHS Cancer Plan states that the government believes that the ultimate goal should be to offer patients a maximum one month wait from an urgent referral for suspected cancer to the beginning of treatment (Department of Health, 2000). Currently lung cancer teams within England are working toward a target of achieving diagnosis within 31 days of the decision to refer and a further 31 days to receiving first treatment (62 days in total).

Coordinated care is a fundamental need for all patients and those with lung cancer, when asked, strongly endorsed this need (Krishnasamy, 2000). It has been suggested that coordinating care and navigating patients through their cancer journey is part of the cancer nurse specialist's role (NHS Executive 1998; Department of Health, 2000). Many nurses, having acknowledged the value of coordinated care, have adopted this as part of their daily practice. However, more recently there have been 'lung tracker' posts developed across the UK. This administrative and clerical post works alongside the lung cancer medical and nursing team and is responsible for tracking patients along their cancer journey, pre-booking appointments and generally organising all hospital visits.

Diagnosis

When diagnosing lung cancer it is preferable to verify the stage of the patient's tumour and also confirm the pathological presence and type of cancer.

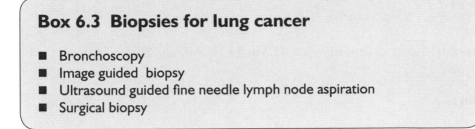

Box 6.3 Biopsies for lung cancer

■ Bronchoscopy
■ Image guided biopsy
■ Ultrasound guided fine needle lymph node aspiration
■ Surgical biopsy

A biopsy can be achieved through a variety of investigations (Box 6.3). This will enable a pathologist to confirm the cancer diagnosis and in most cases differentiate the type of cancer.

Staging

The stage of the cancer describes the size and position of the cancer and whether or not there is evidence that it has invaded adjacent tissues or spread to the lymph nodes or more distant sites. The stage of a lung cancer at presentation has a powerful influence on the prognosis and therefore the choice of treatment.

In non-small cell lung cancer there are broadly four stages (I, II, III, IV) of disease. A systematic approach has been developed to help categorise a patient's disease into one of the four stages. The TNM staging system describes the evidence available regarding an individual's lung cancer disease. 'T' refers the size and location of the primary tumour, 'N' to the involvement of lymph nodes and 'M' refers to the absence (0) or presence (1) of metastases.

The T category is made up of subcategories T1–T4. Increasing number from 1 to 4 represents increasing size and local invasion by the primary tumour. Nodal stages are divided into N1, N2 and N3. The M stage is described as 0 where no metastases are present or 1 if they are. The TNM system allows classification into one of the four stages of disease.

Stage I

All Stage I lesions are completely contained within the lung without evidence of nodal or distant metastatic involvement. Stage IA is classified as T1 N0 M0 or T2 N0 M0, based upon a significantly better 5 year survival outcome.

Stage II

Stage II disease is defined as T1 N1 M0,T2 N1 M0 and T3 N0 M0

Stage III

The Stage III classification is subdivided into IIIA and IIIB. This distinction is important because it differentiates surgical resectability. Stage IIIA patients are considered to be resectable, but Stage IIIB patients are not.

Stage IIIA patients are classified as either T3 N1 M0, or T1–3 N2 M0.

Stage IIIB patients are classified as either T1–3 N3 M0 or T4 N0–3 M0.

Stage IV

Stage IV is defined by any metastatic involvement. These patients are classified as M1 with any T and any N.

To determine the stage of the cancer a variety of investigations or procedures are used (Box 6.4). Positron emission tomography (PET) is used with increasing frequency in the diagnosis of lung cancer.

PET uses a technique that visualises the differences in metabolism of different tissues. Lung cancer cells have a higher rate of metabolism and uptake of glucose than non-cancerous cells, and as a result the indication for using PET in the diagnosis and staging of lung cancer is increasing (Vansteenkiste and Stoobants, 2001). Despite this, access to PET scanning facilities throughout the UK is limited, and patients often have to travel to specialist centres.

A less invasive procedure involves ultrasound of the neck to locate enlarged lymph nodes, followed by fine needle aspiration cytology in patients

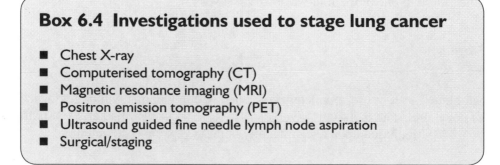

Box 6.4 Investigations used to stage lung cancer

- Chest X-ray
- Computerised tomography (CT)
- Magnetic resonance imaging (MRI)
- Positron emission tomography (PET)
- Ultrasound guided fine needle lymph node aspiration
- Surgical/staging

with suspected lung cancer (Entwisle *et al.*, 2004). If positive, this technique helps to prove the stage of disease, having demonstrated spread from the lung neoplasm to lymph nodes outside of the thorax, and provides a cytology diagnosis.

Types of lung cancer

There are two main categories of lung cancer: non-small cell lung cancer (NSCLC) and small cell lung cancer (SCLC). Of people diagnosed in the UK with lung cancer, 75% to 80% have non-small cell lung cancer, making it the most common type of lung cancer. Only 15% to 20% of people diagnosed with lung cancer have small cell lung cancer.

Non-small cell lung cancer (NSCLC)

There are three major subtypes of non-small cell lung cancer based on the appearance of their cells under the microscope:

- Adenocarcinoma
- Squamous cell carcinoma
- Large cell undifferentiated carcinoma

Cure for NSCLC may be possible with surgery, if detected at an early stage.

Small cell lung cancer (SCLC)

Small cell lung cancer (also called 'oat cell' because SCLC cells have the appearance of oat grains) is a more aggressive type of lung cancer than NSCLC. As stated earlier, SCLC is also less common than NSCLC.

It spreads to the lymph nodes and other organs more quickly than NSCLC, and has commonly spread by the time of diagnosis and is considered a systemic disease at that time.

Treatment

It is important to assess a patient's fitness and general performance prior to deciding a treatment plan (Table 6.1). Depending on the type and stage of the disease and if the patient is reasonably fit (Eastern Co-operative Oncology Group (ECOG) performance status 0–2 – see Table 6.1), they are likely to be offered surgery, chemotherapy, radiotherapy or a combination of these.

Non-small cell lung cancer when diagnosed in the early stages can be cured with surgical resection alone. However most patients present with disease in a more advanced stage. The aim of treatment with more advanced disease is to improve the patient's symptoms, to make them feel better and improve their quality of life. Some patients do live longer as a result of the treatment but this is not the primary aim of the treatment.

Small cell lung cancer is less common. This tumour cell type is far more receptive to the effects of chemotherapy and radiotherapy, and as a result it readily responds to treatment; patients not only experience symptom relief, but also benefit from a measurable improvement in survival.

Table 6.1 ECOG performance status. These scales and criteria are used to assess how the disease affects the daily living abilities of the patient, and determine appropriate treatment and prognosis (Oken et al., 1982).

Grade	ECOG
0	Fully active, able to carry on all pre-disease performance without restriction
1	Restricted in physically strenuous activity but ambulatory and able to carry out work of a light or sedentary nature, e.g. light housework, office work
2	Ambulatory and capable of all self care, but unable to carry out any work activities. Up and about more than 50% of waking hours
3	Capable of only limited self care, confined to bed or chair more than 50% of waking hours
4	Completely disabled. Cannot carry on any self care. Totally confined to bed or chair
5	Dead

Survival

There has been little progress in the treatments available for lung cancer, and five-year survival remains low at 6% for both men and women (Cancer Research UK, 2005).

Numerous studies have found that patients with lung cancer have inequitable access to clinical expertise across the UK as a result of ageism or geographical location (Fergusson *et al.*, 2003; Peake *et al.*, 2003; Melling *et al.*, 2002). Specialist management results in better outcomes for patients. All patients should be referred to a specialist team, regardless of their circumstances or location.

Poor survival rates for lung cancer are in part due to the lack of appropriate treatment. However, research funding for lung cancer, despite its high incidence and mortality, has been poor. In 2002 the National Cancer Research Institute (NCRI) provided insight into cancer research spending within the UK – lung cancer received just 3% of all the government and charity funds available.

If measurable improvements are to be made it is essential that research and development are identified as priorities. Clinical trials are central to the research and development process and are the only reliable way to find out whether a different operation, chemotherapy agent or radiotherapy regime is better than what is already available.

Practical points

- Whilst our understanding of and treatments for lung cancer have improved over the years, there are still inequalities in access and treatment.
- Early diagnosis and treatment are essential.
- Good multidisciplinary management is essential.

References

British Thoracic Society (1998) BTS recommendation to respiratory physicians for organising the care of patients with lung cancer. *Thorax*, **53**(suppl. 1), S1–8.

Brogden, C. (1998) Women and cancer. *Journal of Intravenous Nursing*, **6**, 344–55.

Cancer Research UK (2005) Web site: http://www.cancerresearchuk.org/.

Entwisle *et al.* (2004) Supraclavicular lymph node fine needle aspiration under ultrasound guidance for lung cancer staging. *Poster presentation*, British Thoracic Oncology Group Annual Conference, January.

Fergusson, R. J., Thomsòn, C. S., Brewster, D. H., Brown, P. H. and Milroy, R. (2003) Lung cancer: the importance of seeing a respiratory physician. *European Respiratory Journal*, **21**, 606–10.

Vansteenkiste, J. F. and Stroobants, S. G. (2001) The role of positron emission tomography with F-fluoro-2-deoxy-D-glucose in respiratory oncology. *European Respiratory Journal*, **17**, 802–20.

Krishnasamy, M. (2000) Perceptions of health care need in lung cancer. *Palliative Medicine*, **14**, 410–18.

Melling, P. P., Hatfield, A. C., Muers, M. F., Peake, M. D., Storer, C. J., Round, C. E., Haward, R. A. and Crawford, S. M. (2002) Lung cancer referral patterns in the former Yorkshire region of the UK. *British Journal of Cancer*, **86**, 26–42.

NHS Executive (1998) *Guidance on Commissioning Cancer Services. Improving Outcomes in Lung Cancer: the Manual.* NHS Executive, London.

Department of Health (2000). *The NHS Cancer Plan: a Plan for Investment, a Plan for Reform.* Department of Health, London.

Oken, M. M., Creech, R. H., Tormey, D. C., Horton, J., Davis, T. E., McFadden, E. T. and Carbone, P. P. (1982) Toxicity and response criteria of the Eastern Cooperative Oncology Group. *American Journal of Clinical Oncology*, **5**, 649–55.

Patel, J. D., Bach, P. B. and Kris, M. G. (2004) Lung cancer in US women. *Journal of the American Medical Association*, **291**, 1763–8.

Peake, M. D., Thompson, S., Lowe, D. and Pearson, M. G. (2003) Ageism in the management of lung cancer. *Age and Ageing*, **32**, 171–7.

CHAPTER 7

Diffuse parenchymal lung disease

Jane E. Scullion

The term *diffuse parenchymal lung disease* refers to a broad category of lung diseases, sometimes also referred to as interstitial lung diseases, rather than referring to a single disease entity. These diseases are often grouped together because they have similarities in their clinical presentation, radiographic changes and physiological features (Sullivan and Brown, 1999). Many of them are caused by injury to the lung, which results in chronic inflammation and ultimately leads to progressive scarring known as fibrosis. It is therefore useful to remember that although these diseases have similarities they also have a variety of aetiologies, treatments and prognoses.

Presentation

The patient with diffuse parenchymal lung disease (DPLD) often presents with chronic progressive dyspnoea on exertion and a cough which is often non-productive. There may also be symptoms of underlying connective tissue disease, such as joint pains, erythema and swelling of the joints of the hands, indicative of rheumatoid arthritis, and this may or may not have been previously diagnosed.

Clinical findings

On examination, bilateral inspiratory 'rales' may be heard at the bases of the lungs. Wheeze is not often a presenting symptom unless there is also underly-

Box 7.1 List of some of the common causes of DPLD

- **Occupational related**

Asbestosis
Silicosis
Pneumoconiosis
Hard metal fibrosis
Berylliosis
Talc pneumoconiosis

- **Allergic reactions**

- **Connective tissue disease**

Rheumatoid arthritis
Scleroderma
Systemic lupus erythematosus
Ankylosing spondylitis
Mixed connective tissue disease
Sjogren's syndrome

- **Idiopathic**

Idiopathic pulmonary fibrosis/cryptogenic fibrosing alveolitis
Sarcoidosis
Bronchioitis obliterans organising pneumonia (BOOP)
Adult respiratory distress syndrome (ARDS)
Inflammatory bowel disease
Hepatic cirrhosis
Neurofibromatosis
Lymphangioleiomyomatosis (LAM)
Respiratory bronchiolitis

- **Drug-induced**

Antibiotics	Nitrofurantoin
	Sulfasalazine
Anti-inflammatory agents	Gold
	Aspirin
	Penicillamine
	Methotrexate
Cardiovascular	Amiodarone
	Tocainide
Chemotherapeutic	Bleomycin
	Mitomycin-C

Bulsulfan
Cyclophosphamide
Azathioprine
Methotrexate
Etoposide
Vinblastine
Illicit drugs   Heroin
                       Methadone
Other agents   Talc
                       Isoniazid
                       Oxygen
                       Radiation

This is not an exhaustive list. For a more extensive list please refer to the original document. Modified from Schwarz, M. I. (1993) Clinical review of interstitial lung disease. In: *Interstitial Lung Disease*, 2nd edn (eds. M. I. Schwarz and T. E. King). Mosby, St Louis.

ing airways disease, although in sarcoidosis wheeze may be symptomatic of airways involvement.

Clubbing of the digits is common in DPLD in the latter stages of the disease (Figure 7.1).

Also, in the latter stages of the disease there may be evidence of pulmonary hypertension and right ventricular dysfunction, which may present as oedema of the lower extremities.

Examination may also reveal underlying connective tissue disease: joint inflammation, joint deformities, muscle weakness or skin rash.

It is important to take a comprehensive history from any patient presenting with DPLD in order to ascertain any exposure that could have led to the problem. However, often no causative agent is found.

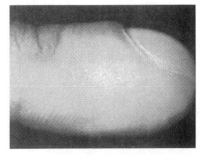

Figure 7.1 Clubbing of the finger, showing loss of vascularity in the nail bed.

Chest X-ray

Although chest X-ray appearance can vary between the various diseases there are often bilateral reticular or reticulonodular opacities and generalised smaller lung volumes. Disease involvement and volume loss are often more prevalent in the bases of the lungs and this may make the hilar regions appear closer to the diaphragm than on a normal X-ray. If there is calcification along the pleura this may be suggestive of asbestos exposure. In the latter stages of the disease process multiple small cysts may be apparent, reflecting end-stage fibrosis and often referred to as 'honeycombing'. CT scans will often demonstrate the peripheral nature of the disease.

Spirometry

The DPLDs are by nature restrictive, so the pattern seen on spirometry is of reduced FEV_1 and FVC but with a preserved FEV_1/FVC ratio. As the alveolar–capillary interface is abnormal the lungs' diffusing capacity for carbon monoxide is decreased. This results in stiff, poorly compliant lungs, which leads eventually to hypoxaemia as the disease develops.

The common DPLD

Asbestosis

This is the consequence of exposure to asbestos, often many years before the patient presents with symptoms, which results in scaring of the lung parenchyma. Often the presentation is with dyspnoea on exertion, and often crackles will be heard on examination. The chest X-ray will show bilateral lower zone reticulonodular infiltrates and there may be pleural plaques. Asking about asbestos exposure is important, but often patients are unable to recall this occurring.

Chronic hypersensitivity pneumonia

Chronic hypersensitivity pneumonitis (CHP) is commonly cause by exposure to organic antigens such as mouldy hay (farmer's lung), animal proteins (common in pigeon fancier's/bird fancier's lung), fungi (mushroom picker's lung), bacteria, and chemicals, such as isocynates. Patients often develop progressive shortness of breath, and it is often more common in non-smokers than smokers. Chest X-ray shows bilateral reticulonodular infiltrates, which may be in the upper lobes. The patient's environmental history is important to ascertain exposure. CHP often responds well to systemic corticosteroids.

Silicosis

Requires exposure to silica over many years and can present in an acute and accelerated form when the exposure is more intense. The occupations in which silica is a likely causative agent are mining, tunnelling, foundary work and sand blasting. A chest X-ray often shows upper zone small nodular opacities which may merge together. There may also be enlargement and calcification of the hilar lymph nodes. Some patients have very few symptoms and may only have minor impairment on lung function testing.

Pneumoconiosis

This develops as a consequence of chronic inhalation of coal dust. There may be multiple small opacities on the chest X-ray, but the patient is often asymptomatic unless they develop progressive fibrosis.

Drug-induced

If the disease is drug-induced it may resolve on cessation of the offending agent, but occasionally systemic corticosteroids are needed.

Idiopathic pulmonary fibrosis/cryptogenic fibrosing alveolitis (IPF/CFA)

This is one of the commonest diseases in this category. It is most common in patients in their 50s to 70s, and there may in some cases be a family history, although often there is no familial link. It is also one of the lung diseases that does not have a casual link with tobacco smoking. Patients with IPF develop progressive dyspnoea on exertion and a non-productive cough. There may be slowly progressive disease before a diagnosis is possible. There are relatively few treatments, with around 50% of patients responding either physiologically or subjectively to prednisolone, azathioprine, cyclophosphamide or colchicines. However, this often merely slows disease progression and the median survival is around 3–5 years from diagnosis.

Sarcoidosis

This is an idiopathic multisystemic inflammatory disorder which commonly involves the lung, although not every patient will have lung involvement. There is a characteristic inflammatory process where the inflammatory cells collect in microscopic nodules known as granulomas. Unlike the other IPF/CFA it is more common in young adults and may spontaneously resolve or follow a benign course. Patients may often be asymptomatic, but abnormalities may be incidental and found on chest X-ray, showing bilateral hilar lymphadenopathy without parenchymal opacities. Systemic corticosteroids are used in symptomatic patients commonly for cough, chest pain, wheezing and dyspnoea.

Therapeutic options

Corticosteroids

These are often the treatment of choice for many types of DPLD and vasculitides. As the diseases demonstrate an uncontrolled inflammatory process, an anti-inflammatory seems a logical choice, but not all patients respond to this treatment and the side-effects can often be as problematic to the patient as the effects of treatment. There is little evidence for length of treatment and this will vary from a few weeks or months to a few years, depending on response to treatment. As individual responses to treatment vary, patients require monitoring for responses to treatment and side-effects.

Cytotoxic agents

A variety of cytotoxic medications have been tried in the management of DPLD. These include azathioprine, cyclosporine and cyclophosphamide, and they all have anti-inflammatory properties and are considered more potent than steroids. The problem with these agents is that the side-effects include depression of the immune system, so patients require close monitoring

Colchicine

This is an antifibrotic medicine that has been used previously to treat gout and may be a useful treatment for DPLDs.

Oxygen therapy

As the result of many DPLDs is hypoxaemia, oxygen therapy is widely used in the treatment, although there is little evidence of its benefits. It is recommended that oxygen is given for generalised hypoxaemia, and hypoxia on exercise and during sleep if clinically indicated. Maintenance of a patient's oxygen levels prevents secondary hypertension and the development of cor pulmonale. It may be that patients will benefit from oxygen at an earlier stage than would be considered necessary on a formal oxygen assessment.

Rehabilitation

Although not extensively studied as a distinct group, rehabilitation may help in maintaining fitness levels for these patients.

Transplantation

This is a last resort for end-stage disease, although there are problems with availability of organs and the fact that in the connective tissue disorders the outcome of transplantation is not as good as in other diseases. Patients may also have concomitant disease, which would exclude them from this option.

Prognosis

For many patients with DPLD the disease is progressive leading to end-stage disease and eventually death. Unfortunately, there are currently few available treatments and these often only result in temporary improvement or slower progression of the disease. However, other possible causes of increasing dyspnoea should be considered in treatment (Box 7.2).

Box 7.2 Possible causes of increasing dyspnoea

- Superimposed infection
- Muscle weakness/osteoporosis due to steroid therapy
- Pulmonary embolism
- Lung cancer
- Atherosclerotic vascular disease

Key points

- This is a diverse group of illnesses, and the diseases have varied aetiology, treatment and prognosis.
- Presenting symptoms are often progressive breathlessness on exertion and cough.
- Lung function usually gives a restrictive pattern.
- Treatments include corticosteroids, cytotoxic agents and oxygen.
- Unfortunately, treatment and care for many of these disease entities is essentially palliative.

Reference

Sullivan, E. J. and Brown, K. K. (1999) Interstitial lung disease. In: *Egan's Fundamentals of Respiratory Care*, 7th edn (eds. C. L. Scanlan, R. L. Wilkins and J. K. Stoller). Mosby, St Louis.

CHAPTER 8

Mesothelioma

Liz Darlison

Introduction

Whilst mesothelioma is not lung cancer, it usually involves the thoracic cavity and patients with the disease are therefore often managed by the lung cancer multidisciplinary team. Mesothelioma is a fatal malignant disease of mesothelial membranes. Principally it affects the pleura and peritoneum, but can also occur in the pericardial pleura and testis.

Pleural mesothelioma causes the pleura to thicken. This thickening of the pleura might begin to press onto the lungs or attach itself to the inside of the chest wall (Figure 8.1). In either case the expansion of the lung becomes progressively restricted by the tumour. A pleural effusion commonly occurs and sometimes several litres can collect between the two layers of the pleura; this affects the lungs' ability to expand and causes the person to feel breathless.

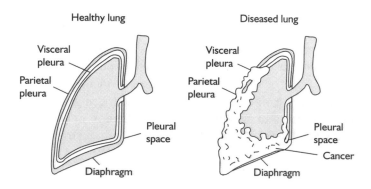

Figure 8.1 Mesothelioma (http://www.mesotheliomacenter.org/).

The peritoneum also has two layers: the inner (visceral) layer, which is next to the abdominal organs, and the outer (parietal) layer, which lines the abdominal wall. Peritoneal mesothelioma causes the peritoneum to thicken and often causes ascites.

Incidence

In the UK just over 2000 people a year are diagnosed with mesothelioma (Cancer Research UK, 2005) and there is approximately one case of peritoneal mesothelioma to every 12 cases of pleural mesothelioma. Peto *et al.* (2005) have predicted that there will continue to be an annual increase in the number of mesothelioma victims. The peak in numbers is expected to be around 1,950–2,450 deaths per year and this will occur between 2011 and 2015.

Survival

Most patients diagnosed with mesothelioma die within 18 months (Clayson, 2003). The range in median survival is reported by Stewart *et al.* (2004) as being 4–18 months, depending on which paper is read. Sadly, this dismal prognosis is also accompanied in many cases by a range of physical symptoms, particularly chest pain and breathlessness, that are difficult to palliate.

Symptoms

Pleural and peritoneal mesothelioma can both cause general symptoms, such as sweating, tiredness, loss of appetite and weight loss. Pleural mesothelioma typically causes patients to feel breathless and/or experience chest pain.

Breathlessness may be due to a combination of factors. The pleura being thickened can act like a rind around the lung, restricting its movement and preventing the lung from expanding. A pleural effusion may also accumulate in the space between the two layers of the pleura, again restricting lung expansion.

Causes

The first epidemiological evidence linking asbestos exposure to the development of mesothelioma was published more that 40 years ago. Stewart *et al.* (2004) explain that currently it is accepted that around 80% of people who develop mesothelioma have had occupational or environmental exposure to asbestos.

It can take many years after being exposed to asbestos for mesothelioma to occur. The length of time taken is referred to as the latency period. Peto *et al.* (2005) report that this is rarely less than 15 years and often exceeds 60 years.

Histological diagnosis

In planning treatment for this disease, especially where clinical trials are involved, it is vital that an accurate diagnosis be achieved. It is sometimes possible to make a cytological diagnosis through fluid drained from the pleural effusion. However, in most cases a definitive diagnosis can only be made following a pleural biopsy.

There are three cell types: epithelioid, sarcomatoid and mixed or biphasic. There is a clear survival benefit associated with the epithelial type.

Staging

Mesothelioma is a difficult cancer to stage. Radiological techniques, chest X-ray and computerised tomography (CT) of the chest and upper abdomen are often used in the first instance, followed if necessary by surgical intervention.

When diagnosing cancer it is necessary to know the type of cancer (e.g. mesothelioma) and also the extent (stage) of the disease. The stage describes the size and position of the cancer and whether or not there is evidence that it has spread to nearby tissues or to other, more distant, sites. Staging can be helpful in assessing prognosis, in making recommendations for treatment and in assessing and comparing the results of treatment.

There are different systems available for staging mesothelioma. The most commonly used system, based on TNM assessment is the International Mesothelioma Interest Group (IMIG) staging system:

- **STAGE 1** Disease limited to the pleura only on one side of the chest.
- **STAGE 2** Disease limited to the pleura on one side of the chest, but the cancer cells have extended from the pleura into the underlying lung tissue or muscle of the diaphragm.
- **STAGE 3** The cancer has spread beyond the pleura to glands in the chest and/or has advanced deeper into the tissues surrounding the pleura.
- **STAGE 4** The cancer has spread to distant organs or tissues or invaded deeply into tissues close to the pleura, e.g. across the diaphragm into the abdomen, into the pleura of the opposite lung or into the spine or heart muscle.

Treatment

The treatment of mesothelioma will depend on a number of things, including the type of mesothelioma, how advanced the disease is, the general health and fitness of the patient and their personal preferences.

There are various treatments that may be recommended for mesothelioma. These include active symptom control, radiotherapy, chemotherapy and surgery. A patient may have just one of these types of treatment or a combination of them. All treatment modalities are considered palliative.

References

Cancer Research UK (2005) Web site: http://www.cancerresearchuk.org/.

Clayson, H. (2003) Suffering in mesothelioma: concepts and contexts. *European Journal of Palliative Care*, **11**(5), 251–5.

Peto, J., Hodgson, J., McElvenny, D., Darnton, A. and Price, M. (2005) The expected burden of mesothelioma mortality in Great Britain from 2002 to 2050. *British Journal of Cancer*, **92**, 587–93.

Stewart, D., Edwards, J., Smythe, R., Waller, D. and O'Byrne, K. (2004) Malignant pleural mesothelioma – an update. *International Journal of Environmental Health*, **10**(1), 26–39.

CHAPTER 9

Oxygen therapy

Ivy Rushby

Introduction

In August 1774 Joseph Priestley focused sunlight through a lens to heat a sample of mercuric oxide (red calx). The resulting gas supported the burning of a candle with a vigorous flame and kept a mouse alive under glass for some time (Woodrow Wilson National Fellowship Foundation, 1992). Priestley declared that he had 'discovered an air five or six times as good as common air' and he called this gas phlogiston. In 1779, it was renamed oxygen by the father of modern chemistry Antoine Lavoisier (Partington, 1989). Whilst some patients believe oxygen to be a better or purer type of air this is not strictly true; oxygen is a pure gas and when used it is important to note that it can be toxic and have side-effects.

What we do know is that oxygen is essential for life. All body tissues need oxygen to survive. Some lung diseases, for example chronic obstructive pulmonary disease (COPD) or interstitial lung disease (fibrotic conditions), can reduce lung function to such an extent that supplemental oxygen is required to maintain normal bodily function.

When oxygen therapy is provided it should be to correct hypoxaemia (deficiency of oxygen in arterial blood) and prevent hypoxia (a lack of oxygen to the tissues, which will result in cell death) (Bateman and Leach, 1998). It is not a treatment for breathlessness unless there is also hypoxaemia, although this is not always understood by patients and some health care professionals.

The aim of this chapter is to extend your knowledge of oxygen therapy in terms of the process of respiration, what goes wrong, when to give supplemental oxygen, how much to give and how it is prescribed. This chapter also covers the assessment for oxygen and care of the patient on long-term oxygen therapy (LTOT).

Respiration

The functions of the lungs are to:

- take in oxygen from the air and transfer it into the blood for use in the tissues of the body
- receive carbon dioxide, the waste product of metabolism, from the blood and excrete it back into the air

Respiration is controlled by the respiratory centre in the medulla in the brain. This centre normally controls respiration by detecting raised carbon dioxide levels in the blood. However with some lung diseases, particularly COPD, there may be a reduction in the excretion of carbon dioxide and the body adapts to a higher carbon dioxide level. If this is insidious the respiratory centre 'switches off' this high carbon dioxide drive and uses low levels of oxygen in the blood to drive respiration. If a patient who is responding to low oxygen levels as a driver for respiration is given a high concentration of oxygen to overcome breathlessness, the patient's drive to breathe might fail and the patient can become drowsy and may even have a respiratory arrest. This means that for patients with COPD low levels of oxygen should be given to keep their oxygen saturations around 90%. In patients with asthma during an asthma attack hypoxaemia can cause death, and these patients need high flow oxygen.

The body relies on the processes of ventilation, gas exchange and circulation to deliver oxygen to the tissues.

Ventilation

A number of diseases can contribute to inadequate ventilation associated with respiratory illness, such as COPD, asthma and pneumonia. Obstructive lung disease causes lung tissue to become thicker and the bronchi and bronchioles to narrow, with loss of elasticity. Less oxygen is transported over the capillary–alveolar interface, the reduced elasticity causes the bronchi and bronchioles to become less compliant, and less air reaches the lungs. Increased secretions may further reduce the diameter of, and even block, the airways.

Although patients with COPD mainly have problems with obstruction, they may have other respiratory problems which may respond to treatments, so it is important to consider all possible causes of shortness of breath and treat optimally.

Gas exchange

Gas exchange in patients is inhibited by damage to the lungs. In COPD this is usually caused by cigarette smoking, although there may be other factors such as occupation, genetics or exposure to harmful toxins.

Circulation

Oxygen is carried around the body in the blood. Around 3% is dissolved in the plasma and 97% is carried as oxyhaemoglobin, which is oxygen bound to haemoglobin in the red blood cells. Haemoglobin is a compound of iron (haem) and four polypeptide chains (globin). Each globin chain is attached to one iron atom. These atoms can carry four molecules of oxygen, and each molecule has two atoms of oxygen. So with four sites to carry oxygen and each site carrying two oxygen atoms this is a very efficient means of carrying oxygen around the body. Each gram of haemoglobin can carry 1.34 ml of oxygen.

Patients with anaemia have less haemoglobin to carry oxygen and, therefore, lower oxygen levels. Patients with some lung diseases can be malnourished and may be anaemic. These patients may compensate for low oxygen levels by increasing their red blood cells so that more oxygen can be transported to the tissues (polycythaemia).

Respiratory failure

Respiratory failure can be defined as an inability to maintain blood gases within normal limits. The decisive measures of pulmonary efficiency are the levels of oxygen and carbon dioxide (CO_2) found in the arterial blood. Whilst oxygen levels can be assessed with a pulse oximeter this does not give any indication of the carbon dioxide level, so this can be difficult to assess in general practice.

Arterial blood gases

These are blood gases taken through an arterial stab and give accurate indications of the level of oxygen and carbon dioxide in the body. This process can be particularly painful for patients, and some centres will undertake ear lobe capillary sampling, which is regarded as accurate and less painful for the patient.

Pulse oximetry

Oxygen saturations can be assessed with the use of a pulse oximeter. In health, normal values for oxygen saturations would be 95% upwards. Readings of 90–92% merit further investigation and those below 90% are usually for cause for concern (Woodrow, 1999). The patient's medical history should be taken into consideration. If a COPD patient has oxygen saturations of 85%, this may be normal for that person and any consideration of giving oxygen should be weighed against the patient's wishes and how they feel (Woodrow, 1999).

The pulse oximeter uses an infrared light to measure both pulse rate and the saturation of haemoglobin – cold hands, with less peripheral blood circulation, give a lower reading and nail polish may prevent the infrared light penetrating the tissues.

Pulse oximeters are accurate at normal levels. However, a number of studies have shown that they become inaccurate with severe hypoxia (Chiappini *et al.*, 1998; Carter *et al.*, 1998).

A pulse oximeter will show oxygen saturations, but not CO_2 levels. It is important to know the CO_2 levels because some patients may have hypercapnia (an increased amount of CO_2 in the blood caused by over-stimulation of the respiratory centre), so the amount of oxygen that can be given will be limited.

In heavy smokers some of the haemoglobin sites will carry carbon monoxide as carboxyhaemoglobin, therefore reducing the amount of oxygen being transported. A pulse oximeter will read this as saturated haemoglobin and give a normal oxygen saturation reading. Despite the normal reading, hypoxia can still be present.

Respiratory failure

There are two types of respiratory failure.

Type I respiratory failure

This occurs when hypoxaemia is present without hypercapnia – the oxygen level in the blood is low and the CO_2 level is within normal limits.

Table 9.1 Some causes of type I respiratory failure.

Asthma	Chest injury
COPD	Thromboembolic pulmonary hyper-
Pulmonary fibrosing	tension
Pneumonia	Lymphatic carcinomatosis
Pneumothorax	Pneumoconiosis
Pulmonary embolism	Granulomatous lung disease
Bronchiectasis	Cyanotic congenital heart disease
Adult respiratory distress syndrome	Fat embolism
Kyphoscoliosis	

Most of the time pulmonary and cardiac causes of respiratory failure lead to hypoxaemia without hypercapnia. This is termed type I respiratory failure (some causes of type I respiratory failure are listed in Table 9.1) (Macnee, 2000).

When the partial pressure of oxygen is normal, but the carrying capacity of the blood is reduced, as a result, for example, of carbon monoxide poisoning or anaemia, the tissues will receive less oxygen.

Type I respiratory failure can be treated using:

- oxygen therapy
- medication to treat the underlying cause of respiratory failure and thereby improve ventilation

Type II respiratory failure

This occurs when hypoxaemia is present together with hypercapnia – the oxygen level in the blood is low and the CO_2 level is raised.

Type II respiratory failure occurs as a result of hypoventilation – the $PaCO_2$ rises and the PaO_2 falls as a result (some causes of type II respiratory failure are listed in Table 9.2). The most common cause is an acute exacerbation of COPD (Macnee, 2000).

Type II respiratory failure can be treated using:

- oxygen therapy titrated to the blood gases or oygen saturations
- medication to treat the underlying causes of respiratory failure
- respiratory stimulants
- non-invasive ventilation

Table 9.2 Some causes of type II respiratory failure.

COPD	Head and cervical cord injury
Asthma	Primary alveolar hypoventilation
Drug overdose	Sleep apnoea
Poisoning	Pulmonary oedema
Myasthenia gravis	ARDS
Polyneuropathy	Myxoedema
Poliomyelitis	Tetanus
Porphyria	Laryngeal oedema
Cervical cordotomy	Foreign body

Often, after the patient has received treatment and has had time to recover, the blood gases can return to normal. This is why oxygen given after an acute event should be a temporary measure and the patient given an oxygen assessment when they are in a stable condition.

Long-term oxygen therapy (LTOT)

The aim of LTOT is to improve the lives of severely hypoxaemic patients (National Institutes of Health, National Heart, Lung and Blood Institute, 2001). LTOT provides significant benefits for a selected group of patients with COPD (Department of Health and Social Security, 1985).

Two major randomised controlled trials, conducted by Nocturnal Oxygen Therapy Trial Group (NOTT) and the Medical Research Council (MRC), have demonstrated that patients with hypoxaemia, caused by respiratory disease, had improved survival rates if they used oxygen for at least 15 hours per day (Nocturnal Oxygen Therapy Trial Group, 1980; Medical Research Council Working Party, 1981). These RCTs informed the development of the Royal College of Physicians guidelines for the prescription and administration of oxygen (see Table 9.3).

Why LTOT helps these patients is unclear, but it has been shown to:

- reduce symptoms of cor pulmonale
- have a psychological benefit
- help prevent cardiac arrhythmia
- reduce polycythaemia
- improve quality of sleep.

(National Institutes of Health, National Heart, Lung and Blood Institute, 2001; Esmond and Mikelsons, 2001)

Table 9.3 Guidelines for the prescription and administration of oxygen.

- COPD with PaO_2 < 7.3 kPa when stable
- COPD with PaO_2 7.3–8 kPa in the presence of polycythaemia, nocturnal hypoxaemia, peripheral oedema or evidence of pulmonary hypertension
- Interstitial lung disease with PaO_2 < 8 kPa and inpatients with PaO_2 > 8 kPa with disabling dyspnoea
- Cystic fibrosis when PaO_2 < 7.3 kPa or PaO_2 7.3–8 kPa in the presence of secondary polycythaemia, nocturnal hypoxaemia, pulmonary hypertension or peripheral oedema
- Pulmonary hypertension without parenchymal lung involvement PaO_2 < 8 kPa
- Neuromuscular or skeletal disorders
- Obstructive sleep apnoea despite continuous positive airways pressure therapy
- Pulmonary malignancy
- Heart failure with daytime PaO_2 < 7.3 kPa or with nocturnal hypoxaemia
- Paediatric respiratory problems

The main complication of oxygen therapy in patients with COPD is hypercapnia if the flow rates are not titrated to the patient's needs.

Potential hazards of oxygen therapy include:

- fire
- oxygen toxicity

Oxygen is potentially a drug and should be ordered and administered as such (Esmond and Mikelsons, 2001; Nursing and Midwifery Council, 2002; British National Formulary, 2006).

Assessment and ordering of oxygen

Before LTOT is ordered the patient must be properly assessed and already be taking optimal medication to control the condition causing hypoxaemia (Medical Research Council Working Party, 1981).

Table 9.4 Indications for the prescription of LTOT.

- PaO_2 from 7.3–8 kPa on air when stable over four weeks or more together with:
  - polycythaemia
  - peripheral oedema suggesting congestive cardiac failure
  - pulmonary hypertension
- Palliation to relieve shortness of breath
- Frequent use of cylinders (> 8 hours per day)

The assessment for LTOT involves two arterial blood gas tests, the second being undertaken three weeks after the first, during a time of clinical stability. LTOT will be ordered if it is indicated from the blood gases (see Table 9.4) (British National Formulary, 2006).

Practical point

Many patients are discharged from hospital with oxygen, but their low levels of oxygen may be an acute feature and as they recover their oxygen levels will return to normal. This is why oxygen levels should be assessed when the patient is stable, otherwise oxygen is an unnecessary treatment modality.

Administration of oxygen

Oxygen therapy can be delivered in three ways:

- Compressed oxygen gas via oxygen cylinders
- Compressed oxygen gas via an oxygen concentrator
- Liquid oxygen via a small lightweight canister

LTOT is usually provided using an oxygen concentrator and is given via a mask or nasal cannulae. It is significantly cheaper to provide LTOT this way, rather than by oxygen cylinders and may be a safer option (Godden and Douglas, 2000).

Depending on how accurate the delivery of oxygen to the patient needs to be there are two delivery systems:

■ fixed performance devices
■ variable performance devices

Fixed performance devices

These delivery systems use the venturi valve and principle of jet mixing. When oxygen passes through a narrow orifice it produces a high-velocity stream that draws in a constant proportion of room air through the venturi valve. The jet mixing can be accurately controlled to give rates of 24–60% oxygen. The masks used with fixed performance devices are large with large holes to allow the escape of carbon dioxide. Fixed performance devices are recommended for patients with type II respiratory failure (Bateman and Leach, 1998). These patients would normally be given 24–28% until blood gas testing is available.

Variable performance devices

These delivery systems use nasal cannulae and masks without a venturi adaptor. The percentage of oxygen delivered depends on the patient's rate and depth of breathing. Variable performance devices are recommended for patients with type I respiratory failure, surgical patients or patients at home with an oxygen concentrator. Due to the risk of hypercapnia, patients with COPD should not be given more than 24–28% oxygen unless blood gases can be assessed (Bateman and Leach, 1998). Oxygen concentrators will normally deliver from one litre to four litres of oxygen. Two litres of oxygen is approximately 24% and four litres of oxygen 28%, dependent on rate and depth of breathing. Humidification is not normally required for these low flow rates, but as oxygen is drying to the mucous membrane, humidification may be prescribed for high flow rates (Bateman and Leach, 1998). High flow rate concentrators can be ordered for patients requiring higher flows of oxygen, often those patients with interstitial lung disease, or two or more concentrators can be 'piggy-backed' together to achieve the desired flow rate.

Although LTOT has been shown to be the only treatment that prolongs the lives of patients with COPD (Nocturnal Oxygen Therapy Trial Group, 1980), to be attached to an oxygen concentrator for 15 hours a day can be restricting. The best time to use the oxygen is overnight. The MRC trial showed that hypoxic patients were more likely to die at night than during the day (Medical Research Council Working Party, 1981). Patients should be encouraged to use oxygen overnight and then to make up their hours in the day. This then allows them time off oxygen to get on with their lives. Being slightly low in oxygen is not as detrimental as patient inactivity.

Changes to LTOT prescriptions

From April 2006 the provision of oxygen changed from prescription only to an ordering system in England and Wales. In Scotland similar arrangements were already in place. From April 2006 oxygen has been ordered via a Home Oxygen Order Form (HOOF). The amount of oxygen required (hours per day) and the flow rate need to be specified by the health care professional. The supplier then determines the appropriate equipment to provide for the patient. The clinician should obtain the patient's consent to pass on patient details to the oxygen supply company and also the fire service. The oxygen supply company will arrange with the patient a time and date to fit the equipment and educate the patient in usage.

The HOOF form should be faxed to the oxygen company with a copy to the PCT and a copy for the patient's notes. The supplier will continue to provide the service requested until a revised order or confirmation that the patient no longer requires a home oxygen service is received.

The companies will be required to provide:

- oxygen concentrators and fittings
- a 24 hour call out service for concentrators
- regular servicing for concentrators
- oxygen cylinders, both large and small, for ambulatory or short burst oxygen
- conservation devices, unless contraindicated. These prolong the life of an ambulatory cylinder as they are triggered when a patient breathes and do not provide a constant flow rate
- liquid oxygen for those who qualify
- other sundry items: masks, nasal cannulae, tubing etc.
- a contact number for emergencies

Community pharmacists may still hold small stocks of oxygen mainly for palliation.

The changes to the service were made on the recommendation of the Department of Health to ensure that patients requiring oxygen receive it with follow-up and assessment, and patients not requiring oxygen would not receive it.

Ambulatory oxygen

A number of studies have demonstrated an improved quality of life and improved exercise tolerance for some patients with COPD if they use ambulatory oxygen (Revill *et al.*, 2000; Eaton *et al.*, 2002). Ambulatory oxygen will maintain oxygen saturations during exercise in those who de-saturate (Nandi *et al.*, 2003). Lightweight portable oxygen cylinders are now available on prescription, and these last approximately four hours when used at a rate of two litres per minute.

Short burst oxygen therapy

Many patients have been prescribed short burst oxygen therapy (SBOT) using a cylinder with occasional 'puffs' of their oxygen. There is currently no evidence to support this practice and oxygen is clearly a treatment for hypoxia, not breathlessness. A patient's medical treatment should be optimised and advice on dealing with breathlessness given. Alternative face cooling methods such as fan therapy may help. Whilst SBOT is not recommended, for some patients there is an obvious placebo effect and if the patient is in the palliative stages of their disease it would be unethical not to palliate symptoms.

Role of the nurse

Patients need a great deal of support when using oxygen, although it is well tolerated and most patients are compliant (Restrick *et al.*, 1993). Some of the most common problems are:

- *Nasal discomfort* – a constant flow of air into the nasal cavity can cause drying of the nasal mucosa and, occasionally, minor bleeding. Patients need to be reassured that, as the nose becomes adapted to the oxygen, this will decrease. If the problem persists, a water-based emollient can be applied.
- *Ear discomfort* – LTOT is usually given via nasal cannulae that are wrapped around the ears, so ears can become sore. A soft piece of gauze or purpose-made ear guards will help, but the discomfort is usually short-lived.
- *Sleep disturbance* – when used at night, the noise of the oxygen concentrator can disturb sleep. Patients need to be advised about where to position the concentrator to minimise disturbance.
- *Restricted movement* – the company providing the concentrator will provide 50 feet of tubing at each outlet point (usually one upstairs and one downstairs), which allows the patient to move about as much as possible.

Table 9.5 Frequently asked questions.

Q	*How is it decided how much oxygen I require?*
A	Usually by taking blood samples, normally as an outpatient.
Q	*Will I become addicted to oxygen?*
A	Patients are only given the amount of oxygen they need. It is in no way addictive.
Q	*How many years will I need it for?*
A	Some patients are given supplementary oxygen temporarily via cylinders; others need oxygen on a more permanent basis via an oxygen concentrator.
Q	*How does the concentrator work?*
A	An oxygen concentrator is an electrical device that draws in room air, separates the oxygen and delivers it to the patient.
Q	*What do I do if visitors want to smoke?*
A	Explain your need for oxygen and ask them either not to smoke or to do it outside.
Q	*Is enough oxygen left in the room for my family to breathe?*
A	Regardless of whether a concentrator is operating or not the oxygen concentration in the room remains the same.
Q	*Is the concentrator oxygen clean enough for me to breathe?*
A	A concentrator has a series of filters and sieve beds to remove dust and trap bacteria.
Q	*Can I cook whilst I am on my oxygen?*
A	Electrical stoves or microwave ovens are no problem. Using supplementary oxygen near an open flame is not recommended.
Q	*Do cylinders and a concentrator give the same oxygen?*
A	Yes. It may feel like there is not as much oxygen from the concentrator as a cylinder. A concentrator delivers oxygen at a lower pressure, but the concentration is the same.

- *Mucosal drying* – anecdotal evidence suggests that drinking plenty or sucking sweets seems to help stimulate salivary glands in the mouth.
- *Drying of respiratory secretions* – anecdotally evidence suggests that nebulised normal saline moistens respiratory secretions, which helps chest clearance.

Some questions frequently asked by patients can be seen in Table 9.5.

Travel with oxygen

It is possible for patients on LTOT to travel, but trips need to be planned. The British Lung Foundation advises:

- plan in advance – never leave things to the last minute
- be realistic – places visited in the past may not be suitable now
- shop around – talk to a number of travel agents as prices and special needs differ
- ask questions – travel companies are used to dealing with special requirements. Ask what you can reasonably expect of them.

Flying with respiratory disease

Commercial aeroplanes fly with a cabin pressure of around 15% oxygen compared to that at sea level. This means that someone with reduced oxygen saturations will be even more compromised than they are at sea level. The BTS standards of care committee points out that these people are at risk from respiratory complications brought about by immobility, dehydration and hypoxaemia (British Thoracic Society, 2002). People with a history of respiratory disease and those hospitalised within six weeks of travelling should be assessed prior to flying. Others who report previous symptoms such as dyspnoea, chest pain, confusion or co-morbid conditions worsened by hypoxaemia, such as cerebral-vascular accident or coronary heart disease, should be assessed before flying. Morgan (2002) points out that patients with a resting oxygen saturation below 92% or 92–95% on air are recommended to take a formal hypoxic challenge test to assess their ability to compensate for altitude pressure. Those with arterial oxygen pressure below 6.6 kPa are urged to make arrangements for supplemental in-flight oxygen. Cramer *et al.* (1996) found that most hypoxaemic patients oxygen saturations returned to within normal limits if given 2 litres of oxygen in flight.

Many schedule airlines will provide in-flight oxygen. However in a study in the USA Stoller *et al.* (1999) found that of 33 airlines contacted, both USA internal and international, there was great variation in:

- cost
- equipment provided
- litres of oxygen available
- information required
- time of booking prior to the flight

(For comprehensive travel information for patients on oxygen therapy see the British Lung Foundation web site www.lunguk.org.)

Use of oxygen in emergencies

Jo Hargrave

In the emergency situation where the patient experiences acute hypoxaemia, priority must be given to maintaining adequate oxygenation of the patient. Emergency oxygen delivery is typically at rates of 10–15 litres/minute. The aim of this is to restore and maintain arterial oxygen levels to ensure tissue oxygenation. This is essential for continued cellular activity. Tissue hypoxia will result in cell death.

The causes of acute hypoxaemia are varied and could be seen in any area of an acute setting. Some examples are listed below:

- Acute asthma
- Cardio-respiratory arrest
- Hypovolaemia
- Mucous plugging
- Myocardial infarction
- Pneumothorax
- Pneumonia
- Pulmonary embolus
- Sedation

Oxygen delivery is dependent on the patient's airway. The ability of patients to maintain their own airway must be assessed. In the self-ventilating patient delivery devices typically include a non-rebreather mask with reservoir. Oxygen is usually delivered at 15 litres/minute through this device. Alternately, the venturi system will be used. This incorporates a fixed rate mask and valve to deliver a predetermined percentage of oxygen. In an emergency situation this would typically be 60%. The patient breathes this in via the mask, and exhaled gases are eliminated via the mask.

In the patient who cannot self-ventilate a bag–valve–mask device with reservoir will be used in association with an artificial airway such as a Guedel airway, or endo-tracheal tube. Fifteen litres/minute of oxygen will be delivered via this circuit and will deliver 85–90% oxygen. The exhaled gases are eliminated via a one-way valve on the mask.

There is widespread concern amongst nurses about the risk of harm to the COPD patient from receiving too much oxygen (Bateman and Leach, 1998; Small and Barsby, 2000). This concern is related to the hypoxic drive of COPD: that is, low levels of oxygen drive the respiratory system in certain lung diseases. The concern is that by delivering a high percentage of oxygen to COPD patients their respiratory drive will be reduced or 'switched off'. Many nurses believe that COPD patients should therefore only be given a maximum of 28% oxygen. In an emergency situation with acute hypoxaemia this will not be adequate. It should be remembered that hypoxic patients need oxygen to avoid cell death (Woodrow, 2004). In reality, only 10–15% of patients with COPD may experience respiratory depression if given more than 28% oxygen, but it is perhaps better in these patients to titrate oxygen saturations to 90% and above (Bateman and Leach, 1998).

In an emergency situation oxygen therapy is often initiated by nursing staff who may be the first to identify an acute deterioration. As nurses we have a professional responsibility to act in our patients' best interests (Woodrow, 2004) and initiate life-saving intervention. However it should be remembered that oxygen therapy is a drug and should be respected as such. Urgent medical attention should be sought, and monitoring commenced of the patient, including pulse oximetry and respiratory rates. Close visual observation should be maintained. Following medical review, arterial blood gases will be taken and the results used to determine the need and level for continuing oxygen therapy. It is likely that this would occur alongside investigation and treatment of the underlying cause of this acute episode.

Conclusion

Oxygen therapy is beneficial to many patients, particularly those who have respiratory disease, but care must be taken when administering it to patients. The costs of providing domiciliary oxygen are high and it is important that patients are carefully assessed before oxygen therapy is prescribed and are monitored thereafter to ensure that they derive physiological and symptomatic benefit from this intervention (Nandi et al., 2003; UK Prescription Pricing Authority, 2002). Oxygen is a drug – there are clear indications for its ordering and guidelines for its administration. As nurses we need to ensure that we are sufficiently knowledgeable about oxygen therapy in order to provide the correct administration of oxygen and also provide support and advice to patients who require such treatments.

Useful web sites

Action on Smoking and Health (ASH): http://www.ash.org.uk/
Provides comprehensive information and analysis of smoking and health-related problems, as well as advice and support for people who want to give up smoking.
Association of Respiratory Nurse Specialists: http://www.arns.co.uk/
Provides useful information for all nurses caring for respiratory patients.
British Lung Foundation: http://www.lunguk.org/
Exists to provide a complete package of support for people living with lung disease and the people who look after them, in hospital and at home.
British Thoracic Society: http://www.brit-thoracic.org.uk/
Provides access to guidelines, reports and patient information on respiratory diseases.
Giving Up Smoking: http://www.givingupsmoking.co.uk/
Provides information and support individuals need to give up smoking for good.
Global Initiative for Chronic Obstructive Lung Disease (GOLD): http://www.gold-copd.com/
Provides up-to-date information on the implementation of the global strategy for the diagnosis, management and prevention of COPD and access to GOLD documents and resources.
National Asthma and Respiratory Training Centre: http://www.nartc.org.uk/
Provides accredited education and training in respiratory and allergic disease for health professionals.
Respiratory Education and Training Centres: http://www.respiratoryetc.com/
Offers a broad spectrum of respiratory courses for health care professionals in both primary and secondary care.
Smoking Cessation: http://www.smoking-cessation.org/
Provides information about a number of smoking cessation therapies and treatment options to help smokers quit successfully.

References

Barnes, P. J. (1999) *Managing Chronic Obstructive Disease*. Science Press, London.
Bateman, N. T. and Leach, R. M. (1998) ABC of oxygen. Acute oxygen therapy. *British Medical Journal*, **317**, 798–801.
British National Formulary (2006) March, 168–9,
British Thoracic Society (2002) Statement on recommendations for managing passengers with respiratory disease who are planning to travel by air. *Thorax*, **57**, 1–2.
Carter, B. G., Carlin, J. B., Tibballs, J., Mead, H., Hochmann, M. and Osborne, A. (1998) Accuracy of two pulse oximeters at low arterial haemoglobin-oxygen saturation. *Critical Care Medicine*, **26**(6), 1128–33.

Chiappini, F., Fuso, L. and Pistelli, R. (1998) Accuracy of a pulse oximeter in the measurement of the oxyhaemoglobin saturation. *European Respiratory Journal*, **11**(3), 716–19.

Cramer, D., Ward, S. and Geddes, D. (1996) Assessment of oxygen supplementation during air travel. *Thorax*, **51**(2), 202–3.

Department of Health and Social Security (1985) *Guidelines for Prescribing Long-Term Oxygen*. National Health Service England and Wales: amendments to drug tariff. DTA/1Z. Department of Health and Social Security, London.

Eaton, T., Garrett, J. E., Young, P., Fergusson, W., Kolbe, J., Rudkin, S. and Whyte, K. (2002) Ambulatory oxygen improves quality of life of COPD patients: a randomised controlled study. *European Respiratory Journal*, **20**(2), 306–12.

Esmond, G. and Mikelsons, C. (2001) Oxygen therapy. In: *Respiratory Nursing* (ed. G. Esmond). Baillière Tindall, London.

Godden, D. J. and Douglas, A. (2000) Indications for referral to secondary care. In: *Clinician's Manual on Chronic Obstructive Pulmonary Disease*. Science Press, London.

MacNee, W. (2000) Respiratory failure. In: *Crofton and Douglas's Respiratory Disease*, 5th edn (eds. A. Seaton, D. Seaton and A. Gordon Leitch). Blackwell Science, Oxford.

Medical Research Council Working Party (1981) Long-term domiciliary oxygen therapy in chronic hypoxia cor pulmonale complicating chronic bronchitis and emphysema. *Lancet*, **I**, 681–6.

Morgan, M. D. L. (2002) *British Medical Journal*, **325**, 1186–7.

Nandi, K., Smith, A. A. and Crawford, K. D. (2003) Oxygen supplementation before or after submaximal exercise in patients with chronic obstructive pulmonary disease. *Thorax*, **58**, 670–3.

National Institutes of Health, National Heart, Lung and Blood Institute (2001) *Global Strategy for the Diagnosis, Management and Prevention of Chronic Obstructive Disease*. NHLBI/WHO Workshop report, Publication number 2701. National Institutes of Health, Bethesda, MD. Also available online at http://www.gold-copd.com/.

Nocturnal Oxygen Therapy Trial Group (1980) Continuous or nocturnal oxygen therapy in hypoxaemic chronic obstructive lung disease. *Annals of Internal Medicine*, **93**, 391–8.

Nursing and Midwifery Council (2002) *Code of Professional Conduct*. Nursing and Midwifery Council, London.

Partington, J. R. (1989) *A Short History of Chemistry*, 3rd edn. Dover, New York.

Restrick, L. J., Paul, W. A., Braid, G. M., Cullinan, P., Moore-Gillon, J. and Wedzicha, J. A. (1993) Assessment and follow up of patients prescribed long-term oxygen treatment. *Thorax*, **48**(7), 7708–13.

Revill, S. M., Singh, S. J. and Morgan, M. D. L. (2000) Randomised controlled trial of ambulatory oxygen and ambulatory ventilator on endurance exercise in COPD. *Respiratory Medicine*, **94**(8), 778–83.

Royal College of Physicians (1999) *Domiciliary Oxygen Therapy Services: Clinical Guidelines and Advice for Prescribes*. Royal College of Physicians, London.

Stoller, J., Hoisington, E. and Auger, G. (1999) A comparative analysis of arranging in flight oxygen aboard commercial air carriers. *Chest*, **115**(4), 991–5.

CHAPTER 10

Pulmonary embolism

Alison Conway

Introduction

An average district general hospital will diagnose 50 cases of pulmonary embolism (PE) annually (Anderson *et al.*, 1991). However, it is thought that the actual numbers of cases may be as high as 1% of all acute emergency admissions, since many pulmonary emboli only become apparent at post mortem (Stein and Henry, 1995).

The aetiology of pulmonary embolism

Most pulmonary emboli arise as detached portions of venous thrombi that have formed in the deep veins of the lower limbs (West, 1998). Other sites include the right side of the heart and the pelvis. Non-thrombotic emboli, such as fat, air and amniotic fluid, may also occur but are rare. In all studies of PE at least one predisposing factor has been found in 80–90% of patients (Lusiani *et al.*, 1996). Factors that predispose to the formation of venous thrombi fall into three broad categories:

- Stasis of blood
- Alterations in the blood coagulation pathway
- Abnormalities of the vessel wall

Table 10.1 shows risk factors for PE (thromboembolic disease) with those in bold being the most common (Donnamaria *et al.*, 1995).

Table 10.1 Risk factors for pulmonary embolism.

Category	Comments
Surgery	**Major abdominal/pelvic surgery** **Hip/knee surgery** Post-operative intensive care
Cardiorespiratory	Acute myocardial infarction Severe respiratory disease
Obstetrics	Pregnancy/puerperium
Lower limb	**Fracture** Varicose veins Stroke/spinal cord injury
Malignant disease	Abdominal/pelvic Metastatic/advanced disease Chemotherapy
Miscellaneous	Increasing age **Previous thrombotic disease** Immobility > 1 week Clotting disorders Trauma Air travel Oral oestrogens Central venous catheters Dehydration Smoking Obesity Family history of thromboembolic disease

Clinical features

The most common clinical features of PE include dyspnoea, tachypnoea (> 20 bpm), pleuritic pain, sense of impending doom, tachycardia, cough, haemoptysis, leg pain and clinical DVT. Although the presence of certain clinical features may not establish the diagnosis of PE, their absence makes a diagnosis of PE extremely unlikely. A number of studies have demonstrated that dyspnoea and tachypnoea are present in 90% of cases. These two, with the presence of pleuritic chest pain, are present in 97%, and the remainder have either chest X-ray changes or low arterial oxygen tension (Stein *et al.*, 1991a).

Investigations

Investigations for PE include some or all of the following.

Chest X-ray

Changes in PE may be fairly non-specific or indeed absent. Chest X-ray findings include segmental collapse, raised hemi-diaphragm, pleural effusion, absence of vascular markings and focal infiltration. The chest X-ray is also useful in excluding other causes of dyspnoea, such as left ventricular failure, pneumothorax, pneumonia or lung cancer.

Ventilation/perfusion (VQ) scanning

This involves the intravenous injection of a radioisotope and the inhalation of a different radioisotope to compare the ratio of ventilation to perfusion. VQ scanning should normally be performed within 24 hours of onset of symptoms consistent with PE. Many scans revert to normal quite rapidly and over half do so within one week (British Thoracic Society, 1997).

Scans must be reported within the clinical context of the presentation and in conjunction with a recent good-quality chest X-ray.

Although a high-probability VQ scan correctly identifies pulmonary embolism in up to 92% of patients with clinical suspicion of PE, they have some limitations (PIOPED, 1990). The interpretation of VQ scans may be misleading or difficult in the presence of a number of respiratory diseases, including previous PE, COPD, lung fibrosis and proximal lung tumours. Left ventricular failure can also cause localised variations in pulmonary perfusion. In these situations computerised tomography (CT) scanning with pulmonary angiography is ideally used.

ECG

ECG changes in PE are quite common (Stein *et al.*, 1991b), but are often non-specific: for example, tachycardia, atrial fibrillation, and changes in the ST segment and/or T wave. Massive pulmonary emboli may result in signs of right heart strain. Once again the ECG may be useful in excluding or diagnosing other conditions such as pericardial disease or myocardial infarction.

Arterial blood gases

Since pulmonary embolism is characterised by a mismatch of the ventilation/ perfusion ratio it is common to see a physiological shunt, hypoxia and hypocapnia. If the embolus is large enough to cause circulatory collapse a metabolic acidosis may be seen.

Plasma D-dimers

This simple blood test relies on the measurement of cross-linked fibrin degradation, D-dimer. Values are rarely normal (< 200) in those with acute venous thromboembolism. However, D-dimers may also be raised in a number of other situations, including infection and trauma. The value of this test is that if the D-dimers are less than 200 then a diagnosis of PE is highly unlikely.

Management

Anticoagulation remains the mainstay of treatment. Unless contraindicated, heparin should be started if there is a high or moderate suspicion of PE, pending results of further investigations. There are two different forms of heparin preparation commonly used: standard heparin and low molecular weight heparin (LMWH). Standard heparin is given as intravenous infusion beginning with a loading dose of 5,000–10,000 units, followed by an infusion of 400–600 units/ kg daily (British Thoracic Society, 1997). Dosage is titrated against results of activated partial thromboplastin time (APTT) test. This should measure 1.5–2.5 times the control values. Low molecular weight heparin is becoming increasingly used due to its advantages of rapid but predictable anticoagulation, easy subcutaneous administration, set dosage syringes and no requirement for laboratory monitoring. Heparin is continued during the introduction of warfarin, until adequate anticoagulation is achieved.

Heparin may be discontinued once the international normalised ratio (INR) is within the therapeutic range of 2.0–3.0 (British Thoracic Society, 1997). If the risk factors for venous thromboembolism are thought to be temporary, e.g. post surgery, six weeks to three months of anticoagulant treatment is usually sufficient to prevent recurrence. The longer the duration of anticoagulant therapy the greater the benefits in terms of reduced thromboembolism. However, this has to be balanced against the risks of bleeding. As stated, first episodes of

PE will usually only require 3–6 months of treatment. However, in the case of recurrent thromboembolism, lifelong anticoagulation may be necessary.

Thrombolysis (using streptokinase or urokinase), pulmonary embolectomy and inferior vena-caval (IVC) filters are also used in the treatment of pulmonary embolus but these are uncommon and are usually reserved for patients with massive PE (the former two) or recurrent multiple pulmonary emboli (the latter).

Conclusion

PE may well be more common than previously thought due to the relative difficulty in confirming a definite diagnosis, rather than excluding it through current investigative techniques. Clinical assessment of patients and their relative risk factors remains a crucial part in accurate diagnosis and early, appropriate instigation of treatment.

References

Anderson, F. A., Wheeler, H.B., Goldberg, R. J., Hosmer, D. W., Patwardhan, N. A., Jovanovic, B., Forcier, A. and Dalen, J. E. (1991) A population-based perspective of the hospital incidence and case-fatality rates of deep vein thrombosis and pulmonary embolism. *Archives of Internal Medicine*. **151**, 933–8.

British Thoracic Society (1997) Suspected acute pulmonary embolism: a practical approach. *Thorax*, **52**(suppl.), S1–24.

Donnamaria, V., Palla, A., Petruzelli, S., Manganelli, D., Baldi, S. and Giuntini, C. (1995) A way to select, on clinical grounds, patients with high risk for pulmonary embolism: a retrospective analysis in a nested case-control study. *Respiration*, **62**, 201–4.

Lusiani, L., Visona, A., Banonome, A., Persavento, R. and Zanco, P. (1996) The characteristics of the thrombi of lower limbs, as detected by ultrasonic scanning, do not predict pulmonary embolism. *Chest*, **110**, 996–1000.

PIOPED (1990) Value of the ventilation/perfusion scan in acute pulmonary embolism. *Journal of the American Medical Association*, **263**, 2753–9.

Stein, P. D. and Henry, J. W. (1995) Prevalence of acute pulmonary embolism among patients in a general hospital and at autopsy. *Chest*, **108**, 978–81.

Stein, P. D., Saltzman, H. A. and Weg, J. G. (1991a) Clinical characteristics of patients with acute pulmonary embolism. *American Journal of Cardiology*, **68**, 1723–4.

Stein, P. D., Terrin, M. L., Hales, C. A., Palevsky, H. I., Saltzman, H. A., Thompson, B. T. and Weg, J. G. (1991b) Clinical, laboratory, roentgenographic and electrocardiographic findings in patients with acute pulmonary embolism and no pre-existing cardiac or pulmonary disease. *Chest*, **100**, 598–603.

West, J. B. (1998) *Pulmonary Pathophysiology*, 5th edn, pp. 104–10. Williams & Wilkins, Baltimore, MD.

CHAPTER II

Pulmonary function tests

D. D. Vara

Introduction

This chapter gives an overview of the main investigations performed within respiratory physiology departments.

Breathing tests are performed on patients presenting with shortness of breath, or on those with a known respiratory condition in order to monitor progress or therapeutic improvements.

The majority of lung function testing involves the patient breathing into specialist equipment, via a mouthpiece, and measurements of capacity and efficiency are made.

All of the measurements made are compared to predicted normal ranges quoted from the European Community for Coal and Steel (ECCS). The predicted normal range for each patient is dependent on their age, height and sex. (The predicted equations for the basic tests are included in the appendix).

The main tests and services discussed in this chapter are:

- Basic spirometry
- Full pulmonary function testing
- Bronchodilator response
- Blood gases
- Methacholine challenge
- Exercise testing
- Sleep studies
- Nasal ventilation

Various other specialist investigations are also carried out depending on the clinical features of the patient.

Note: Contraindications to pulmonary function testing are listed in the appendix.

Types of lung disease

There are two main categories of lung disease, though some conditions may exhibit characteristics of both.

The tests performed in the respiratory unit help to determine, along with other investigations, whether the patient has either a restrictive or obstructive condition, the severity of the condition and the effectiveness of any treatment given.

Restrictive lung disease

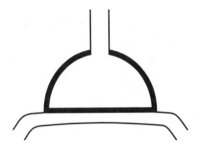

Figure 11.1 Restriction of the lung around the lung.

This category includes lung fibrosis and chest wall deformities. These are conditions that cause a reduction of the lung volume, i.e. the lungs cannot expand fully either from:

■ A stiffening of the lung tissue, reducing elasticity, or
■ A stiffening/deformity of the chest wall, reducing expansion.

Obstructive lung disease

These diseases include asthma and COPD (Chronic Obstructive Pulmonary Disease), a term which encompasses chronic bronchitis and emphysema. These are conditions which cause narrowed airways, either from (Figure 11.3):

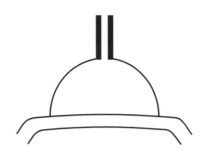

Figure 11.2 Obstructed lung occurring in the airway.

- Excessive mucus in the airway lumen
- Enlarged mucus glands or contracted muscle within the airway wall
- Loss of support from surrounding tissue making the airways 'floppy'

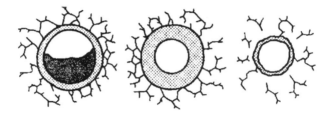

Figure 11.3 Causes of narrowed airways.

Spirometry

What is spirometry?

Spirometry is the measurement of dynamic breathing. It is the most common measurement made in respiratory physiology and gives valuable information on which type of lung disease the patient has.

It involves the patient taking in a big breath in until the lungs are full, and blowing as hard and as fast as they can into the spirometer.

The most common measurements made in spirometry are:

- **PEF – Peak Expiratory Flow** (litres/minute)
The maximal flow achieved from a forced expiration, starting from a position of full inspiration.

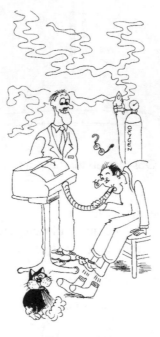

Figure 11.4

This is used to indicate the presence of airflow obstruction (either fixed or variable) in conditions such as COPD and asthma. Serial measurements of PEF may be performed by suspected asthmatics to aid diagnosis, and are often used by known asthmatics to provide an objective indicator of severity of bronchoconstriction.

■ **FEV₁ – Forced Expired Volume in 1 second** (litres)
The volume of air forcibly expelled from the lungs in the first second of the forced blow out, starting from a position of full inspiration.

■ **FVC – Forced Vital Capacity** (litres)
The total volume of air forcibly expelled from the lungs, starting from a position of full inspiration.

■ **FEV₁/FVC ratio**
A ratio of the FEV_1 divided by the FVC, expressed as a percentage, shows how much of the FVC is expired in the first second. If this ratio is less than 72% it suggests a degree of airways obstruction.

These measurements are used to indicate the type of lung disease present (i.e. restrictive or obstructive) and the severity of airflow limitation.

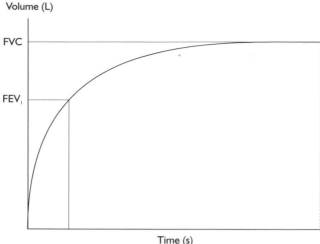

Figure 11.5 A volume/time graph.

How are the measurements displayed?

There are two graphical methods of displaying the spirometry measurement. The first is the simplest, and involves plotting volume expired against time.

A 'normal' volume/time graph is shown in Figure 11.5.

This is the simplest form of spirometry for the patient to perform. It involves the patient blowing out as long and as fast as possible until they are empty.

The graph shows a large change in volume at the start of the blow out, when the lungs are full. After the first second of the blow, the volume expelled relative to time gradually reduces as the lungs empty.

The other method of displaying the spirometry measurement involves plotting flow expired and inspired against volume.

A 'normal' flow/volume loop is shown in Figure 11.6.

This form of spirometry involves the patient blowing out as long and as fast as possible until the lungs are empty, and breathing in as fast as possible until they are full. The graph shows the breath out at the top and the breath in at the bottom.

At the start of the breath out, the flow rate is high, as the lungs are full of air and the airways are open. As the lungs empty the flow rate decreases until all the air is expelled. On the breath in, the flow rate starts off low as the lungs are empty, then increase and decrease again as the lungs fill.

This method is used to distinguish between different types of airflow obstruction, and can show the presence of small airways disease and (from the inspiration) upper airflow obstruction, e.g. due to a goitre.

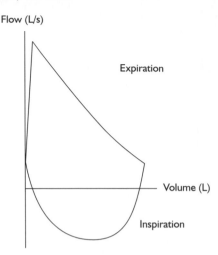

Figure 11.6 A flow/volume loop.

Spirometry results

The spirometry measurement enables the results to be compared with the predicted values for that patient, and to help establish whether a restrictive or obstructive condition is present.

Restrictive lung disease

This will normally result in a reduction in the FEV_1 and FVC.

The PEF may be reduced or within normal limits, while the FEV_1/FVC ratio is usually normal or maybe raised slightly as the lungs are small and empty quickly.

A typical restrictive volume/time trace is shown in Figure 11.7.

A typical restrictive flow/volume loop trace is shown in Figure 11.8. This shows a relatively 'normal shaped' flow/volume loop which is simply a smaller volume than predicted.

Obstructive lung disease

This will normally result in a decreased FEV_1, while the FVC may be normal or reduced.

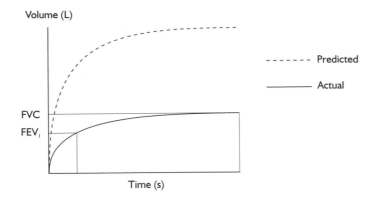

Figure 11.7 A typical restrictive volume/time trace.

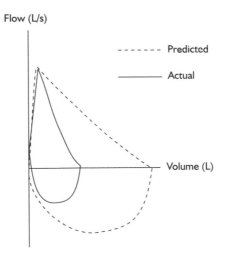

Figure 11.8 A typical restrictive flow/volume loop trace.

Obstruction is differentiated from restriction by a reduced FEV$_1$/FVC ratio. While the PEF is usually reduced, it may be normal in early disease.

The FEV$_1$ is reduced as the airways are narrowed and therefore reduces the rate at which the air can be expelled.

The degree of airflow obstruction may be categorised by the reduction in the FEV$_1$/FVC ratio (ATS Guidelines; National Collaborating Centre for Chronic Conditions, 2004).

FEV$_1$/FVC ratio	60–80%	**= mild airflow obstruction**
FEV$_1$/FVC ratio	40–60%	**= moderate airflow obstruction**
FEV$_1$/FVC ratio	less than 40%	**= severe airflow obstruction**

Practical point

■ NICE guidelines use slightly different categories of disease severity, so be sure you know which ones are being used.

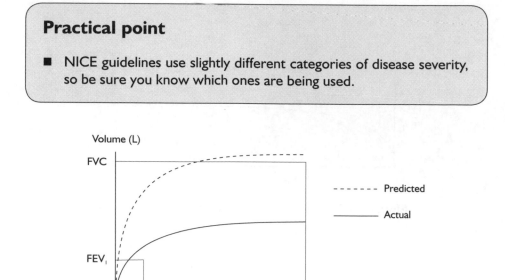

Figure 11.9 A typical obstructive volume/time trace.

A typical obstructive volume/time trace is shown in Figure 11.9.

A typical obstructive flow/volume loop trace is shown in Figure 11.10. This demonstrates a 'normal shaped' inspiration. Only expiration is usually affected in conditions such as COPD. In this case the expiration shows a 'scooped-out'

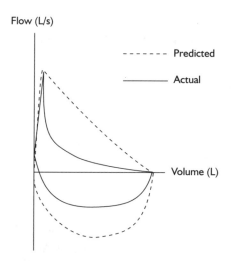

Figure 11.10 A typical obstructive flow/volume loop trace.

appearance as the flow rates reduce as the airways collapse, thus restricting the flow of air.

If a patient suffers with an obstruction in the upper airways, for example due to a goitre, then the inspiration and expiration would be affected. The peak flows of both would be reduced, showing a flattening of the inspiratory and expiratory curves.

Bronchodilator response

Patients found to have a degree of airflow obstruction on their spirometry may be given a dose of inhaled medication to open their airways. The spirometry test may then be repeated to see whether the medication has improved the results.

How does the medication work?

There are two main types of inhaled medication that promote bronchodilation, which and can be used to test the patients in the department. They may be delivered to the patient via Metered Dose Inhaler (MDI) and a spacer device or a nebuliser (which turns a liquid medication into a mist to breathe in).

B_2 *agonists – e.g. salbutamol (Ventolin) or salmetererol (Serevent)*

These are drugs that mimic the activity of the sympathetic nervous system. They stimulate the B_2 receptors in the airway smooth muscle, causing relaxation and therefore bronchodilation.

These work quickly, so the patient's spirometry may be retested 20 minutes after administration.

Anticholinergic – e.g. ipratropium bromide (Atrovent) or oxytropium (Oxis)

These drugs oppose the action of the parasympathetic nervous system. They block the binding site of the neurotransmitter acetylcholine, which prevents bronchoconstriction and therefore results in bronchodilation.

They take slightly longer to take effect, so the patient's spirometry is therefore repeated 45 minutes after administration.

What is classed as a significant response? (British Thoracic Society COPD Guidelines)

A significant response to a bronchodilator drug is classified as either:

- 15% and 200 ml increase in FEV_1
- 15% and 330 ml increase in FVC

Lung volume test

The FRC measurement

This test is used to measure the patient's ventilated lung volume, which can give information on whether the patient's lung volume is reduced (i.e. restricted) or enlarged (i.e. hyper-inflated).

FRC stands for **Functional Residual Capacity**, and is the volume of air remaining in the lungs at the end of a normal breath out (end-tidal breath).

The FRC includes:

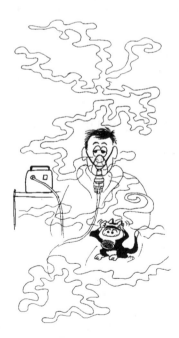

Figure 11.11

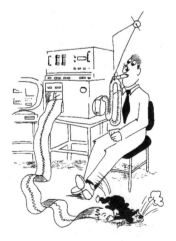

Figure 11.12

- The extra volume of air which can be expelled out of the lungs during a maximal expiration (expiratory reserve volume ERV), and
- The volume of air which remains in the lungs at the end of a maximal expiration (residual volume RV)

As the residual volume cannot be expired from the lungs, it cannot be measured directly. It is therefore measured indirectly by a method called helium dilution.

What is helium dilution?

A mixture of 13% helium is used to obtain a measurement of FRC. Helium is an inert gas that does not transfer across the alveolar membrane.

The FRC is measured by the patient rebreathing through a closed breathing circuit containing the helium mixture for 3–5 min. As the patient rebreathes, the helium dilutes with the patient's FRC.

During the test, the carbon dioxide breathed out by the patient is absorbed by soda lime crystals (to ensure there is no build up), and any oxygen used up is replaced. Once the helium has diluted and reached equilibrium, the volume of FRC can be calculated (see appendix for equation). Note: this test is dependent on there being no leaking of the helium mixture during the test, *and* it is only able to measure well-ventilated lung volume.

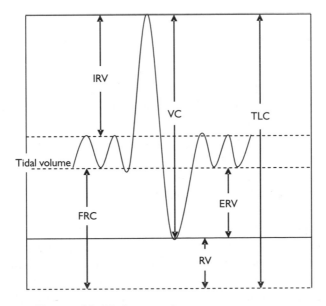

Figure 11.13 Lung volume measurements.

What other measurements are made during the lung volume test?

Once the patient's FRC is measured, the patient is asked to perform some relaxed vital capacity manoeuvres (RVCs). These involve the patient breathing steadily in until the lungs are full, and steadily out until they are empty.

From these measurements, further subdivisions of lung volumes are calculated, including the total lung capacity.

The measurements made are shown in Figure 11.13.

Lung volume results

The measurements obtained in the FRC test enable the lung volumes to be compared to normal predicted values for that individual. This will help to determine whether they have an obstructive or restrictive condition.

Restrictive lung disease

This will normally result in a general reduction in lung volumes below the normal range. The expansion of the lung is restricted; therefore the lung capacities are reduced. A TLC below 85% predicted is considered restrictive.

Obstructive lung disease

This will generally result in either normal or raised lung volume parameters. Mild COPD and asthma may present with lung volumes within normal limits. Advanced COPD and emphysema may present with raised lung volumes (particularly residual volume (RV)). The lung tissue loses elastic recoil and becomes hyper-inflated.

In emphysema, gas may become trapped behind damaged airways which is suggested by a raised RV/TLC ratio, i.e. a large proportion of the total lung capacity is composed of residual volume (trapped gas).

A TLC greater than 115% predicted is considered hyper-inflated, while an RV/TLC ratio greater than 50% suggests gas trapping.

In these patients other methods of measuring lung volumes may be preferred, such as body plethysmography. This involves the patient performing a test in a sealed unit, and is used to calculate the total volume of gas in the thorax, including that trapped behind collapsed airways.

Transfer factor test (diffusion)

The transfer factor measurement

This test assesses the ability of the lungs to transfer gases from the air breathed in into the blood stream.

The test results obtained depend:

■ Ventilation to the alveolar units
■ Diffusion across the alveolar–capillary membrane, and
■ Perfusion of the lungs

The test uses carbon monoxide (CO) to measure the gas exchange, and is therefore named the carbon monoxide transfer factor or diffusion test.

How does the carbon monoxide test work?

Carbon monoxide is used in the test as it readily combines with haemoglobin, 210 times faster than oxygen, and offers no back tension across the alveoli.

The procedure is:

■ The patient inspires a mixture containing less than 0.3% CO to total lung capacity from an inspiratory bag.
■ The breath is then held for 9 seconds to allow the CO to transfer into the blood stream.
■ The patient then expires into the expiratory bag.

An alveolar sample is taken from the expired bag and measured for CO. This sample is then compared to the inspiratory sample and the transfer factor calculated.

What measurements are made during the test?

TLCO is the measure of the transfer of the lung for carbon monoxide. The transfer coefficient (KCO) determines the ability of each litre of lung volume measured in the test to transfer carbon monoxide.

Transfer factor results

The transfer factor and transfer coefficient are compared with predicted values to determine the type of lung disease present and its severity.

Restrictive lung disease

This will normally result in a general reduction in the transfer factor (TLCO) below the normal range. The expansion of the lung is restricted; therefore the diffusion capability of the lung is reduced.

If the restriction is due to diseases of the alveolar capillary membrane, such as fibrosis (alveolar thickening), then the transfer coefficient (KCO) per lung unit will usually be reduced below the predicted range.

If the restriction is due only to chest wall or diaphragmatic problems (not the lungs) then the KCO will usually be normal or raised.

Obstructive lung disease

In asthma, the TLCO and/or KCO may be raised due to inflammation causing increased perfusion. In mild COPD/bronchitis the TLCO and KCO may be normal, or only the TLCO slightly reduced. In severe COPD with emphysema, the TLCO and KCO are normally both reduced due to the loss of alveolar units, and therefore reduced surface area for gas exchange.

Blood gas analysis (ear-lobe capillary sample)

It is useful in respiratory patients to assess the level of respiratory gases in the blood. This is done by obtaining a sample of arterial blood, which has been newly oxygenated by the lungs.

Arterial blood may be obtained by taking a sample directly from an artery (arterial puncture). This test, however, is quite painful and can cause damage to the artery or cause a blood clot to develop.

An arterialised sample can also be obtained from the capillary bed in the ear-lobe. This is a quick, safe and relatively painless test giving important information on the pulmonary status of the patient.

How is the test performed?

- Vasodilating cream is applied to the ear lobe and left for 5–10 min.
- Once the ear is warm, the cream is removed and the ear lobe cleaned.
- The lower tip is scratched with a scalpel blade tip and the blood sample collected in a capillary tube.
- The capillary sample is then analysed in a blood gas analyser.

What measurements are made during the test?

Unit	Measurement	Normal range
PaO_2	Partial pressure of oxygen	12.66–9.97 kPa
pCO_2	Partial pressure of carbon dioxide	4.5–6.0 kPa
pH	Hydrogen ion concentration	7.35–7.45
HCO_3	Bicarbonate ion concentration	22–24 mmol/L
BE	Base excess	± 2.0 mmol/L
O_2 sat	Oxygen saturation	94–98%

Blood gas results

The measurement of blood gas status may be compared with the normal ranges to determine the severity of lung disease.

In lung disease, patients may become unable to maintain normal levels of respiratory gases in the blood due to the damage to the lungs. If they fall below or above normal limits then this change may be described as:

- **Hypoxaemia**
PaO_2 below normal, which may result in inadequate tissue oxygenation

- **Hypercapnia**
pCO_2 above normal range, which will result if alveolar ventilation cannot keep up with the metabolic demands of the body

In more advanced lung disease, the patient's blood gas status may be affected to a greater degree. This is described as **respiratory failure**, of which there are two types that may occur, depending on the type and level of lung disease.

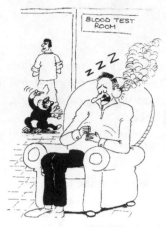

Figure 11.14

Type I respiratory failure

This type of failure is characterised by a PaO_2 less than 8 kPa. Conditions in which type I failure occurs include: early COPD, pulmonary fibrosis, pneumonia or mild asthma.

Type II respiratory failure

Type II failures involve a PaO_2 less than 8 kPa and a pCO_2 greater than 6.5 kPa. Conditions in which type II failure occurs include: COPD with emphysema, longstanding extrapulmonary restriction causing hypoventilation or severe asthma.

Other tests using the blood gas measurement

Ear-lobe capillary samples are also used in other tests within the department.

Long-term oxygen therapy assessment

Patients with hypoxaemia (low PaO_2) may benefit from supplemental oxygen for home use, taken via a cylinder when required.

Patients with a PaO_2 consistently below 8 kPa benefit from long-term oxygen therapy. This involves using supplemental oxygen via an oxygen concentrator, and should be used for at least 16 hours per day.

Within the department, patients are assessed to determine the level of oxygen required to increase their PaO_2 to greater than 8 kPa.

This test involves the patient having an ear-lobe sample taken on two separate visits to the department (to ensure clinical stability). On the second visit they are attached to an oxygen concentrator for 1 hour and the blood gas status is reassessed. The oxygen is increased until the PaO_2 is above 8 kPa.

In-flight assessment

This test assesses whether a patient requires supplemental oxygen on a flight. Inspired oxygen at ground level is 20.9%. In an aircraft cabin this is only 15% due to pressurisation. Patients with lung disease may have difficulty in breathing at a lower inspired oxygen level.

The test involves the patient having a baseline ear-lobe gas sample taken. They then inspire 15% oxygen from a special cylinder (while monitoring oxygen saturation via a finger probe) for 20 min before a repeat ear-lobe sample is taken. If the PaO_2 falls below 6.8 kPa, this would suggest that supplemental oxygen is required when flying.

Methacholine challenge

In patients where asthma is suspected, as the condition is characterised by variable airflow obstruction (hyper-reactive airways), the results on the spirometry measurement may appear normal.

In these cases a methacholine challenge may be performed to determine the stability of the airways.

What does the test involve?

In order to determine whether the patient has hyper-reactive airways, they inhale increasing concentrations of a substance called methacholine. Methacholine is a bronchoconstrictor agent, i.e. it will cause airway narrowing.

In patients with asthma, significant airway narrowing will occur at much lower doses than with non-asthmatics.

The degree of airway narrowing is assessed by measuring the patient's FEV_1 between each increasing dose of methacholine. A drop of 20% from baseline is classed as significant, and if this occurs at a low concentration of methacholine this would suggest a diagnosis of asthma.

Classification of results

The concentration at which the patient's FEV_1 drops by 20% indicates the severity of the airway hyper-reactivity:

Grade	Concentration range
Severe	less than 0.25 mg/ml
Moderate	0.25–2.0 mg/ml
Mild	2.0–8.0 mg/ml
Normal	above 8.0 mg/ml
Possible mild	4.0–16.0 mg/ml

Exercise testing

Different exercise tests are used for different reasons in respiratory physiology.

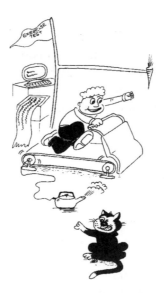

Figure 11.15

Shuttle walking test

This is an incremental exercise test that is used predominantly in rehabilitation programmes. It is used to assess the exercise tolerance of the patient initially, then on repeated tests to assess improvement.

Exercise-induced asthma exercise test

This exercise test involves the measurement of spirometry pre- and post-exercise. A 'steady state' method of exercise is used, which involves maintaining a constant heart rate.

In exercise-induced asthma the patients FEV_1 will drop significantly after exercise (i.e. more thann 20%)

Cardio-respiratory exercise test

This is an incremental exercise test during which the oxygen uptake, oxygen saturation, heart rate and electrocardiogram (ECG) are measured (amongst many other parameters). The test is performed on either a cycle ergometer or treadmill.

This test is used to determine whether the patient's shortness of breath is due to respiratory or cardiac problems, or a combination of both.

Sleep studies

Some respiratory conditions cause a disturbance in the respiratory cycle during sleep. Therefore sleep studies may be performed to help in the diagnosis of sleep disturbance.

Two different sleep studies are performed in the department.

Pulse oximetry

This is a simple sleep study that monitors two parameters while the patient sleeps: oxygen saturation, which is the percentage of haemoglobin that has oxygen bound to it, and heart rate. These are measured via a probe worn over the finger, attached to a monitor around the wrist. The probe uses an infrared light source to detect the level of oxyhaemoglobin. The heart rate is picked up via the pulse.

These recordings indicate whether the oxygen saturation drops (due to respiratory disturbance) or the heart rate rises (due to arousal).

Partial polysomnography

This is a more complex sleep study which measures oxygen saturation and heart rate as before, but also measures chest wall movement, airflow (from the nose and mouth) snore and body position.

These are measured via a monitor worn around the patient's chest and electrodes and sensors stuck to the chest, neck and face.

These recordings indicate whether the patient's breathing slows or stops during sleep. This more detailed study should indicate the cause of saturation dip or heart rate arousal.

Sleep study results

There are two main types of condition that affect the respiratory cycle during sleep, resulting in oxygen saturation dips.

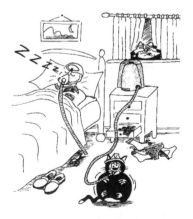

Figure 11.16

Obstructive sleep apnoea (OSA)

This describes an occlusion of the upper airway. If the upper airway is 'floppy', then during sleep it may collapse and prevent airflow. This causes a pause in breathing and therefore a subsequent drop in oxygen level.

This condition will be picked up from oxygen dips on pulse-oximetry, and the pauses in breathing from the partial polysomnography, which is required to diagnose OSA.

The dips in oxygen level and increases in heart rate (due to arousals when overcoming the obstruction) cause tiredness and morning headaches.

Alveolar hypoventilation

This describes a decrease in the rate and depth of breathing, which reduces the ventilation to the alveolar units. If this reduces too much then the lung become unable to maintain normal blood gas levels due to the metabolic demands of the body. This causes a decrease in the oxygen level and an increase in the carbon dioxide level as gas exchange is compromised.

It may occur in patients with chest wall deformity such as kyphoscoliosis, where the respiratory depth and rate drops.

Patients with neuromuscular disease affecting the respiratory muscles may also have dips in oxygen saturation particularly during deep (REM) sleep. During REM sleep all muscles are paralysed except for the diaphragm. Therefore if the diaphragm is affected by a condition then respiration during this deep sleep will be compromised.

CPAP therapy

Treatment for obstructive sleep apnoea (OSA)

There are several treatments for OSA, depending on the underlying cause. Body position modification, weight reduction, oral devices such as a mandibular advancement device or surgery on the upper airway may be considered.

OSA can also be treated by the use of a CPAP machine, which stands for Continuous Positive Airway Pressure. This delivers a stream of air via a mask over the nose to splint the airway open. This course is usually considered first.

The machine needs only to be used at night, when the patient is lying down and the airways are liable to collapse. By preventing the collapse of the airway, the patient's oxygen saturation remains constant, and the symptoms of tiredness and headaches should be relieved.

Nasal ventilation

Nasal ventilation describes a machine similar to a CPAP (described earlier) which uses a nasal mask to deliver air to the patient. Different types of machine are used in the treatment of different conditions.

Treatment for alveolar hypoventilation

Patients who breathe too shallowly or slowly overnight may require a machine to help maintain their normal breathing pattern. The machine is known as a NIPPV, which stands for Non-Invasive Positive Pressure Ventilation.

This machine cycles with the patient's normal breathing pattern by delivering a set pressure or volume when the patient takes a breath, which helps to inflate the patient's lungs. At the end of the breath in, the pressure is removed to allow passive expiration. The machine is also set with a backup rate, so if the patient pauses for too long between breaths the machine will automatically initiate a breath in.

Treatment for exacerbations of COPD

Nasal ventilators are also used in the treatment of chronic obstructive pulmonary disease. These patients are admitted to hospital with a worsening of their breathing, which is often due to a chest infection.

As their breathing worsens, they may not ventilate sufficiently and therefore develop type II respiratory failure or worsen existing respiratory failure (low oxygen and high carbon dioxide). In this case, the patient may require nasal ventilation for a short period of time to support their breathing.

Ventilators used in these conditions are those that provide inspiratory and expiratory support which helps to keep the airways open and improve alveolar ventilation. By increasing the patient's ventilation, the patient's oxygen level should increase and the carbon dioxide level should decrease, thus returning the blood gas status to 'normal', or at least to their previous stable chronic status.

Appendix

The reference equations for calculating the predicted values for spirometry are listed below, for male and female. A refers to age in years; H refers to height in metres.

Male	FEV_1	$4.30H - 0.029A - 2.49$
	FVC	$5.76H - 0.026A - 4.34$
Female	FEV_1	$3.95H - 0.025A - 2.60$

FVC	$4.43H - 0.026A - 2.89$

The equation to calculate FRC by helium dilution is shown below. He_1 and He_2 are the initial and final concentrations of helium, and V_1 is the volume of the circuit.

$$\mathbf{FRC} = V_1 \times (He_1 - He_2)/He_2$$

Contraindications for pulmonary function testing

- Unstable angina
- Recent myocardial Infarction (up to 6 weeks)
- Aortic aneurysm
- Recent thoracic, abdominal or eye surgery
- Haemoptysis of unknown origin
- Pneumothorax
- Pulmonary embolism
- Acute disorder affecting performance, such as nausea or vomiting

Suggested further reading

Respiratory function testing and physiology

Gibson, G. J. (1996) *Clinical Tests of Respiratory Function*. Chapman & Hall, London.

Hughes, J. M. B. and Pride, N. B. (1999) *Lung Function Tests – Physiological Principles and Clinical Applications*. W. B. Saunders, Philadelphia.

Kinnear, W. J. M. (1997) *Lung Function Tests – A Guide to Their Interpretation*. Nottingham University Press, Nottingham.

National Collaborating Centre for Chronic Conditions (2004) Chronic obstructive pulmonary disease; national clinical guidelines for management of chronic obstructive pulmonary disease in adults in primary and secondary care. *Thorax*, **54**(suppl. 1), 1–232.

Nunn, J. F. (1996) *Applied Respiratory Physiology*. Chapman & Hall, London.

West, J. B. (1995) *Respiratory Physiology – the Essentials*, 5th edn. Williams & Wilkins, Baltimore, MD.

West, J. B. (1997) *Pulmonary Pathophysiology – the Essentials*, 5th edn. Williams & Wilkins, Baltimore, MD.

Exercise testing

Jones, N. L. (1988) *Clinical Exercise Testing*, 3rd edn. W. B. Saunders, Philadelphia.

Non-invasive ventilation

Simonds, A. K. (2001) *Non-Invasive Respiratory Support – a Practical Handbook*, 2nd edn. Arnold, London.

Sleep studies

Stradling, J. R. (1993) *Handbook of Sleep-Related Breathing Disorders*. Oxford University Press, Oxford.

CHAPTER 12

Pulmonary rehabilitation

Johanna Williams

Introduction

Pulmonary rehabilitation can be described as being a multidisciplinary programme, consisting of exercise and education, aimed at reducing physical deconditioning and improving the ability of people with chronic lung disease to cope with their condition.

Rehabilitation should be a holistic process where the ultimate aim is to 'restore the individual to the fullest medical, mental, emotional, social and vocational potential of which the person is capable' (Wouters, 2004). Pulmonary rehabilitation (PR) has been defined by the American Thoracic Society as being 'a multidisciplinary programme of care for patients with chronic respiratory impairment that is individually tailored and designed to optimise physical and social performance and autonomy' (American Thoracic Society, 1999).

Most pulmonary rehabilitation programmes in the UK are hospital based, but provision of rehabilitation around the country is inconsistent, with only one respiratory centre in five providing a programme. Where rehabilitation programmes do exist, people with lung disease can gain a lot from networking with others who have the same problems, and group support can provide the motivation to persevere with an exercise programme.

Rationale for pulmonary rehabilitation – the vicious cycle of inactivity

Patients with chronic lung disease tend to become progressively more inactive as their disease progresses. As they become more breathless, everyday tasks

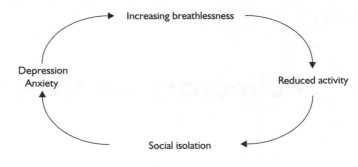

Figure 12.1 The vicious cycle of breathlessness.

such as walking or activities of daily living become more difficult. Over a period of time their level of activity gradually reduces, leading to deconditioning of the cardio-vascular system. Peripheral muscle weakness and deconditioning are also very common, as is malnutrition.

Along with the physical deconditioning that occurs, patients often feel depressed and anxious, which can cause them to restrict their activity due to fear of breathlessness (Figure 12.1). Unfortunately most patients with chronic lung disease only present with their breathlessness when it is having a significant effect on their lives.

Pulmonary rehabilitation aims to reverse this vicious cycle and 'restore patients with debilitating and disabling disease to an optimally functioning state' (Wouters, 2004).

Selection of patients

The British Thoracic Society (BTS) guidelines from (1997) give guidance on which type of patients should be considered for PR:

- The majority of patients seen in PR programmes will have COPD but all patients should be considered who have dyspnoea from respiratory disease (e.g. chronic asthma, bronchiectasis, restrictive lung disease, hyperventilation syndrome, pre-lung surgery, chronic heart failure).
- Disabled by breathlessness (MRC 3–5; see Box 12.1).
- No selection should be made based upon age, impairment, disability or smoking status.

Box 12.1 Medical Research Council (MRC) dyspnoea scale

1   I only get breathless with strenuous exercise
2   I get short of breath when hurrying on the level or walking up a slight hill
3   I walk slower than people of the same age because of breathlessness, or I have to stop for breath when walking at my own pace on the level
4   I stop for breath after walking about 100 yards or after a few minutes on the level
5   I am too breathless to leave the house or I am breathless when dressing or undressing

Box 12.2 Specific exclusion criteria (American College of Sports Medicine, 1991)

- Unstable angina or other recent acute cardiac events
- Uncontrolled ventricular dysrhythmia
- Acute congestive heart failure
- Severe aortic stenosis
- Known or suspected dissecting aneurysm
- Recent systemic or pulmonary embolus
- Resting diastolic blood pressure > 100 mm Hg or resting systolic blood pressure >180 mm Hg

- Consider any significant co-morbidities and how they affect someone's ability to exercise (Box 12.2).
- Consider factors such as poor motivation and logistical factors such as geography, transport, equipment usage and the group composition.

There is increasing evidence that patients with many levels of disease severity will benefit from pulmonary rehabilitation (National Collaborating Centre for Chronic Conditions, 2004), although those that have the motivation to want to improve their lives are likely to do better. While severity of lung function has very little correlation with how disabled someone is by their breathlessness, rehabilitation presumes that anyone experiencing breathlessness is likely to benefit.

Referral for PR is often delayed until a patient has advanced lung disease. Although these patients can derive a lot of benefit from the programme, referral at an earlier stage would enable more preventative strategies to be employed, such as smoking cessation and nutritional therapy, while allowing the patient to maximise the benefits of rehabilitation[1].

Patients should also be optimally managed pharmacologically prior to commencing PR. Patients on oxygen therapy should not be excluded from PR if ambulatory oxygen can be provided.

Aims of PR

The aims of PR are broad and reflect the multidisciplinary approach to patient care:

- To improve exercise tolerance and physical functioning
- To help to control symptoms
- To improve quality of life
- To improve patients' knowledge about their condition and treatment
- To reduce the psychological impact of the disease and resulting disability

Components of PR

Exercise training is a crucial part of the management of COPD. Regular exercise can bring about many beneficial changes in people with chronic lung disease. These include the following:

- Cardio-vascular reconditioning
- Desensitisation to the sensation of breathlessness
- Improved efficiency of the lungs
- Increased muscle strength
- Improved flexibility
- Better balance
- Enhanced body image

In general, exercise training can be divided into two types: endurance (or aerobic) training and strength training.

Aerobic training consists of large muscle activity (e.g. walking or cycling), ideally for a duration of 20–30 minutes performed at least three times a week. The optimal intensity of exercise is subject to debate, but training is normally based on either a percentage of maximal heart rate or percentage of maximal oxygen uptake. Most rehabilitation programmes in the UK offer classes two to three times a week for a varying duration, but commonly for between six to eight weeks.

Strength training is often used in combination with aerobic training and involves the use of either free weights or isokinetic machines. Strength training is increasingly being seen as important in addressing the peripheral muscle weakness that is commonly seen in patients with COPD, but as yet this is an area that still requires further research.

Using the FITT principle (frequency, intensity, type and time), the recommendations below are for an individual with mild to moderate COPD (Table 12.1) (Cooper, 2003).

Exercise is to be encouraged in people with lung disease. The exercise programme should be flexible and individualised to take into account the fluctuations in a person's condition. Any significant change in medical condition requires reassessment of the goals and risks of the exercise programme. The type of exercise to be selected should be one that is enjoyable and improves the person's ability to perform usual daily activities. Walking, cycling, swimming or conditioning exercises such as Pilates or Tai Chi are all suitable.

Table 12.1 Exercise recommendations.

Type	Intensity/frequency/time
Aerobic Large muscle activities such as walking, cycling, swimming	Comfortable pace (monitor breathlessness using Borg scales (Table 12.2; Borg, 1982) 3–7 days/week 30 min/session (shorter intermittent sessions may be necessary initially) Emphasise progression of duration over intensity
Strength Free weights Isotonic/isokinetic machines	Low resistance, high reps\2–3 days/week
Flexibility Stretching	3 sessions/week

Table 12.2 The Borg breathlessness scale.

0	Nothing at all
0.5	Very, very slight
1	Very slight
2	Slight
3	Moderate
4	Somewhat severe
5	Severe
6	
7	Very severe
8	
9	Very, very severe
10	Maximal

Education

Patient education is a central feature of most programmes, but is not effective alone in improving quality of life or physical performance (British Thoracic Society, 1997). The term 'self-management' has become popular when describing interventions designed to maximise concordance with medical advice such as medication, management of exacerbations and the adoption of a healthy lifestyle. The content of the education programme will vary depending on local resources, but areas commonly covered are:

- Disease education (pathology, physiology, oxygen therapy)
- Physiotherapy skills (relaxation, chest clearance techniques, breathing control)
- Nutritional advice
- Management of exacerbations
- Energy conservation
- Benefits of physical exercise
- Psychosocial interventions (anxiety management, coping strategies)

The setting and duration of PR

The majority of PR programmes in the UK have historically taken place in a secondary care setting. However, there are an increasing number of rehabilitation programmes now being delivered in the primary care setting. This has the advantage of the patient being seen locally, eliminating long travelling times to hospital. However, it tends only to be suitable for the lower risk patients, i.e. those not on oxygen or without significant co-morbities such as angina. In parts of Europe, domiciliary rehabilitation has been proven to be effective (Wijkstra *et al.*, 1996), and there is growing interest in delivering rehabilitation in the acute inpatient setting, following an admission to hospital with exacerbation, or shortly after coming out of hospital (Man *et al.*, 2004).

There is still conflicting evidence regarding the optimal duration of PR. In the UK the majority of programmes run for between six and eight weeks, although recent evidence has shown that for some patients a four-week course has been seen to produce similar results in terms of improved exercise tolerance and health-related quality of life to those of patients completing a seven-week course (Green *et al.*, 2001). In parts of Europe, the trend is for patients to come for rehabilitation for a much longer period (usually six months) with advocates claiming that the effect of rehabilitation is more long-lasting (Troosters *et al.*, 2000). Inpatient rehabilitation has been shown to have similar effects to outpatient-based rehabilitation, but is expensive to run, although improvements may occur in a shorter period (Puente-Maestu *et al.*, 2000). Cost comparison suggests that hospital outpatient rehabilitation is currently the most efficient form of delivery (British Thoracic Society, 1997).

In terms of the number of sessions a week needed for rehabilitation to be effective, the most recent BTS guidelines suggest that at least three exercise sessions per week are necessary for sustained improvement. It appears that supervision of some sessions is essential (Puente-Maestu *et al.*, 2000). Therefore, taking a pragmatic approach, the majority of programmes in the UK tend to include two supervised sessions per week, with additional instructions to train at home on a daily basis.

Outcomes of rehabilitation

There is now a large body of research confirming that PR improves exercise capacity. Significant improvements have been documented in terms of walking distance, muscle strength and domestic function (Berry *et al.*, 1999; Ries *et al.*, 1995; Wedzicha *et al.*, 1998; Griffiths *et al.*, 2000). PR also produces significant improvements in health status such as emotional functioning and mastery (the degree of control someone feels they have over their condition). Many studies have shown a reduction in anxiety and depression following PR. Symptoms such as breathlessness significantly decrease and patients report increased satisfaction in how they perform activities of daily living (Sewell *et al.*, 2005; Williams *et al.*, 2003; Finnerty *et al.*, 2001).

A large study examining health care utilisation following a six-week course of PR found that in comparison with a control group who received 'usual care', patients in the rehabilitation group had the same number of hospital admissions but spent only half as long in hospital (10 days versus 21 days). The authors of the study report that PR has been found to be cost-effective and results in financial benefits for the NHS (Griffiths *et al.*, 2000).

National Institute for Clinical Excellence (NICE) Guidelines

National guidelines have recently been published which are likely to have an impact on future provision of PR (National Collaborating Centre for Chronic Conditions, 2004). These guidelines state that:

- PR should be available to all appropriate patients with Chronic Obstructive Respiratory disease (COPD)
- PR should be offered to all patients who consider themselves functionally disabled by COPD (MRC grade 3 and above)
- PR programmes should include multi-component, multidisciplinary interventions and be individually tailored to needs
- The rehabilitation process should incorporate physical training, disease education, nutrition, psychological and behavioural interventions
- Patients should be made aware of the benefits of pulmonary rehabilitation and the commitment required

The future for PR

The NICE guidelines (National Collaborating Centre for Chronic Conditions, 2004) are likely to result in increased provision of PR as more health care professionals and patients become aware of the benefits of rehabilitation and exercise their right to access an intervention that has a strong evidence base. Pulmonary rehabilitation has been proven to be effective in a variety of settings, including hospital inpatient, hospital outpatient, the community and the home. Further research is still needed to determine the optimal duration and setting of rehabilitation and also on how to maintain the improvements gained.

References

Wouters, E. F. M. (2004) Pulmonary rehabilitation. *Breathe*, **1**(1), 33–42.

American Thoracic Society (1999) Pulmonary rehabilitation. American Journal of Respiratory Critical Care Medicine, **159**, 1666–82.

British Thoracic Society (1997) Guidelines on the management of COPD. The BTS standards of care committee. *Thorax*, **52**(suppl. 5), S1–28.

American College of Sports Medicine (1991) *Guidelines for Exercise Testing and Prescription*, 4th edn. Lea & Febiger, Philadelphia.

National Collaborating Centre for Chronic Conditions (2004) Chronic obstructive pulmonary disease; national clinical guidelines for management of chronic obstructive pulmonary disease in adults in primary and secondary care. *Thorax*, **54**(suppl. 1), 1–232.

Cooper, C. B. (2003) Chronic obstructive pulmonary disease. In: *ACSM'S Exercise Management for Persons with Chronic Disease and Disabilities*, 2nd edn (eds. J. I. Durstine and G. E. Moore). Human Kinetics, Champaign, Illinois.

Borg, G. (1982) Psychophysical basis of perceived exertion. *Medicine and Science in Sports and Exercise*, **14**, 377–81.

Wijkstra, P. J., van der Mark, T. W., Kraan, J., van Altena, R., Koëter, G. H. and Postma, D. S. (1996) Effects of home rehabilitation on physical performance in patients with chronic obstructive pulmonary disease (COPD). *European Respiratory Journal*, **9**, 104–10.

Man, W. D. C., Polkey, M. I., Donaldson, N., Gray, B. J. and Moxham, J. (2004) Community pulmonary rehabilitation after hospitalisation for acute exacerbations of chronic obstructive pulmonary disease: randomised controlled study. *British Medical Journal*, **10**, 1136–41.

Green, R. H., Singh, S. J., Williams, J. E. A. and Morgan, M. D. L. (2001) A randomised controlled trial of four weeks versus seven weeks of pulmonary rehabilitation in chronic obstructive pulmonary disease. *Thorax*, **56**(2), 143–5.

Troosters, T., Gosselink, R. and Decramer, M. (2000) Short- and long-term effects of outpatient rehabilitation in patients with chronic obstructive pulmonary disease: a randomized trial. *American Journal of Medicine*, **109**(3), 207–12

Fuchs-Climent, D., Le Gallais, D., Varray, A., Desplan, J., Cadopi, M. and Prefaut, C. (1999) Quality of life and exercise tolerance in chronic obstructive pulmonary disease: effects of a short and intensive inpatient rehabilitation program. *American Journal of Physical Medicine & Rehabilitation*, **78**, 33–5.

Puente-Maestu, L., Sanz, M. L., Sanz, P., Cubillo, J. M., Mayol, J. and Casaburi, R. (2000) Comparison of effects of supervised versus self-monitored training programmes in patients with chronic obstructive pulmonary disease. *European Respiratory Journal*, **15**, 517–25.

Berry, M. J., Rejeski, W. J., Adair, N. E. and Zaccaro, D. (1999) Exercise rehabilitation and chronic obstructive pulmonary disease stage. *American Journal of Respiratory Critical Care Medicine*, **160**, 1248–53.

Ries, A. L., Kaplan, R. M., Limberg, T. M. and Prewitt, L. M. (1995) Effects of pulmonary rehabilitation on physiologic and psychosocial outcomes in patients with chronic obstructive pulmonary disease. *Annals of Internal Medicine*, **122**, 823–32.

Wedzicha, J. A., Bestall, J. C., Garrod, R., Garnham, R. and Jones, P. W. (1998) Randomized controlled trial of pulmonary rehabilitation in severe chronic obstructive pulmonary disease, stratified with the MRC dyspnoea scale. *European Respiratory Journal*, **12**, 363–9.

Griffiths, T. L., Burr, M. L., Campbell, I. A., Lewis-Jenkins, V., Mullins, J., Shiels, K., Turner-Lawlor, P. J., Payne, N., Newcombe, R. G., Lonescu, A. A., Thomas, J. and Tunbridge, J. (2000) Results at 1 year of outpatient multidisciplinary pulmonary rehabilitation; a randomised controlled trial. *Lancet*, **355**, 362–8.

Sewell, L., Singh, S. J., Williams, J. E. A., Collier, R. and Morgan, M. D. L. (2005) Can individualised rehabilitation improve functional independence in elderly patients with COPD? *Chest*, **128**(3), 1194–200.

Williams, J. E. A., Singh, S. J., Sewell, L. and Morgan, M. D. L. (2003) Health status measurement: sensitivity of the self-reported Chronic Respiratory Questionnaire (CRQ-SR) in pulmonary rehabilitation. *Thorax*, **58**, 515–18.

Finnerty, J. P., Keeping, I., Bullough, I. and Jones, J. (2001) The effectiveness of outpatient pulmonary rehabilitation in chronic lung disease. A randomised controlled trial. *Chest*, **119**, 1705–10.

CHAPTER 13

Respiratory assessment

Alison Conway

Respiratory assessment encompasses all aspects of nursing and is an essential tool. Abnormalities in breathing pattern can be due to disease in any system. For example, a patient with a head injury may have a decreased respiratory rate due to rising intracranial pressure. Diabetic ketoacidosis may present with rapid Kussmal's respiration. Musculoskeletal chest pain causes rapid, shallow breathing due to pain and an unwillingness to fully expand the chest. The list of causes for altered breathing pattern is substantial and includes anaemia, shock, cardiac disease, renal acidosis, neurological disease and muscular dysfunction.

It is clear from this list that an accurate assessment of the patient's respiratory status is essential in all disciplines.

General observation

In any setting the general appearance of the patient can provide a wealth of information about the patient's health status, particularly in relation to respiratory disease. Whilst talking to the patient, make an overall observation and consider the following:

- Does the patient look ill?
- Is the patient breathless at rest?
- Is the patient unkempt (implying that dyspnoea is affecting their daily activities)?
- Is the patient in pain?
- Level of consciousness/confusion
- Breathing pattern
- Audible stridor/wheeze
- Cyanosis

- Signs of overt weight loss
- Signs of anaemia/pallor/polycythaemia

Cyanosis

There are two types of cyanosis – peripheral and central – and it is imperative that the two are distinguished correctly, as the presence of central cyanosis is a far more significant clinical sign.

Peripheral cyanosis is the presence of blue extremities, e.g. fingers and toes, but the tongue remains pink. This is commonly seen in healthy people in cold weather, in Raynaud's syndrome and in the presence of peripheral vascular disease.

Central cyanosis is the presence of blue lips and tongue and represents arterial hypoxaemia. For central cyanosis to be present the arterial PaO_2 is less that 8 kPa (SaO_2 of < 85%). Erythropoietin secretion is increased in the presence of chronic hypoxaemia leading to secondary polycythaemia. Cyanosis is only recognisable when at least 5 g/dl of haemoglobin is unsaturated. This explains why cyanosis is more easily recognised in patients with polycythaemia and more difficult to see in anaemic patients.

Finger clubbing

This poorly understood clinical sign is present in a number of respiratory diseases, but also in a number of other systemic disorders (see Table 13.1).

Whilst established finger clubbing is very obvious, early sings of clubbing may be difficult to determine. One key question is whether this is a new

Key point

Finger clubbing *does not* occur in COPD and so should be considered as a potential indicator of an occult pulmonary neoplasm. Patients with COPD are likely to have a significant smoking history and will be over the age of 50. Both are significant risk factors for an increased incidence of pulmonary carcinoma.

Table 13.1 Finger clubbing in various disorders.

Respiratory	Bronchiectasis
	Lung abscess
	Emphysema
	Cystic fibrosis
	Bronchial carcinoma
	Mesothelioma
	Asbestosis
	Cryptogenic fibrosing alveolitis
	Chronic pulmonary tuberculosis
Cardiac	Sub-acute bacterial endocarditis
	Congenital cyanotic heart disease
Gastrointestinal	Primary biliary cirrhosis
	Crohn's disease
	Ulcerative colitis
Congenital	(autosomal dominant)

phenomenon for that patient and how rapidly the alteration in nail shape has occurred. This may help determine the cause of the clubbing.

Clubbing is characterised by the following:

- Loss of angle between the nail bed and the nail
- Increased curvature of the nail
- Increase in the size of the distal phalanx
- Spongy nail bed when depressed (nail bed fluctuance)

Respiratory rate/pattern

This simple, equipment-free test is one of the most useful, instantly available assessment tools for any nurse. It is also the least frequently performed and least accurately performed. In today's technology-overloaded health service, respiratory rate and pattern are a simple, yet vital assessment tool and accurate recording of both can provide a wealth of information on any patient, in any setting (Turner, 2003).

The normal resting respiratory rate of a healthy adult is 12–14 breaths per minute. This is much lower than the 20 breaths per minute that is routinely recorded by many nurses on observation charts. A respiratory rate of above 20 is classed as tachypnoea and is therefore an abnormal result. One of the problems with recording respiratory rate is that it is difficult to conduct without both the patient and the nurse feeling self-conscious about such direct observation.

One of the easiest ways to record respiratory rate is to simultaneously take the patient's pulse. Both pulse and respiration rate should be recorded for a period of at least 30 seconds. If you therefore count the pulse rate for the first 30 seconds and the respiratory rate for the latter half of the minute you can accurately record both observations without the patient being aware of their respiratory pattern being observed. It is very disconcerting to have your chest stared at from the end of the bed, and in response to this intrusion patients will alter their breathing pattern and rate accordingly. By taking the patient's pulse, or at least adopting this familiar, expected task, the patient remains relaxed and is generally unaware of your observation. For even greater accuracy (and comfort for the patient) you can rest their wrist against their abdomen and you are then able to feel the movement of respiration under your hand. If you utilise the methods suggested above, always ensure that the patient's arm is resting either against their abdomen or on the chair/bed, as it is tiring to elevate your arm for this length of time. This is particularly important for patients who are utilising their accessory muscles of respiration.

Respiratory rate is utilised in a number of national guidelines as an indicator of severity (British Thoracic Society, 2004) and accurate recording is imperative.

Respiratory pattern is rarely recorded, but the depth, regularity, symmetry and type of breath should be observed and considered in relation to the patient's history and symptoms. Shallow, rapid breathing may be due to pain, shock, bronchoconstriction, anxiety and a multitude of other causes. Rapid, deep sighing breaths may be in response to metabolic acidosis, e.g. ketoacidosis or renal tubular acidosis. Slow shallow breathing may be due to raised intracranial pressure, overdose, neurological dysfunction or the characteristic Cheyne–Stokes respiration that is usually a precursor to death.

To summarise – this simple, effective, technology-free and quick assessment tool is vital for nurses in any healthcare setting, but is rarely performed, and when done is often performed badly (Breakhall, 2004; Carberry, 2002).

Pulse oximetry

Pulse oximetry is now widely utilised in secondary care in both medical and surgical nursing. It is also becoming increasingly available in primary care, in

Table 13.2 Limiting factors of pulse oximetry.

- Poor peripheral circulation – cold, shock, peripheral vascular disease, Raynaud's syndrome

- Cardiac arrhythmia – tachycardia, bradycardia, SVT, atrial fibrillation

- Anaemia – all the Hb available is fully saturated, but the patient may be hypoxic

- Skin colour – darkly pigmented nails

- Nail varnish

- Position of probe on finger – clubbing, fungal nail infection, severe eczema on nails

- Saturation < 80% – below this figure pulse oximetry becomes inaccurate and a 5% variation either way can occur

walk-in centres and in the ambulance service. It is a relatively cheap, rapid and non-invasive method of estimating arterial oxygenation. It must, however, be interpreted according to the patient and in conjunction with other observations. Pulse oximeters measure the amount of infrared light absorbed by saturated and non-saturated haemoglobin (spectrophotometry) (West, 2000). This gives an estimate of the percentage of saturated haemoglobin, which is an indicator of arterial oxygenation. The infrared light shines onto a capillary bed adjacent to the skin's surface. The most common site is the nail bed of the fingers. However, toes and earlobes may also be used. Pulse oximetry depends on a number of factors to ensure its accuracy, in particular adequate pulsatile blood flow to the peripheries. The other limiting factors of pulse oximetry are shown in Table 13.2.

It is important to note that the main limitation of pulse oximetry is that it does not measure carbon dioxide and so should only be used to give an initial assessment of pulmonary ventilation. If the patient's condition alters or there is a doubt as to whether the patient may have Type II respiratory failure, then arterial blood gas analysis is essential.

Key point

If a patient has an oxygen saturation of 92% or less, arterial blood gas analysis is essential. Due to the sigmoid shape of the oxyhaemoglobin dissociation curve, saturations below 92% signify a rapid fall in partial pressure of oxygen (PaO_2) and accurate assessment of this is vital to prevent tissue hypoxia.

Arterial blood gas analysis

Arterial blood gas analysis is confined to use in secondary care, but is still utilised in a variety of settings. It provides not only an accurate assessment of pulmonary ventilation but also of the acid/base balance of the body. Radial artery puncture is the most common site for this invasive procedure, but brachial and femoral arteries may also be used.

Arterial blood gas analysis gives information on the pH, partial pressure of oxygen (PaO_2), partial pressure of carbon dioxide ($PaCO_2$), the base excess (BE), bicarbonate ion (HCO_3) concentration and the oxygen saturation (SaO_2). The normal ranges for these are shown in Table 13.3.

Blood gases are often poorly understood unless you are familiar with the normal values and are used to interpreting results on a daily basis.

The following is a brief explanation of what all the terms mean in simple terms and in what I hope is an easy to understand format.

pH – a measure of the acidity or alkalinity of arterial blood. Strictly speaking it is a measure of the number of free hydrogen ions; the higher the number of these, the more acidic something is and the lower the pH (pH 7 is neutral, so the body is slightly alkaline). The body's enzyme pathways depend on the maintenance of a very narrow pH band on which to function correctly. If pH shifts outside of these parameters by even a small amount, significant changes occur within the body to try to revert the pH to within normal limits. Receptors in the medulla, aortic and carotid bodies all respond to changes in pH by altering pulmonary ventilation rate and excretion of bicarbonate ions by the kidneys.

Partial pressure of oxygen – the measure of the amount of pressure a gas exerts in a solution, at room temperature and at sea level. In this case we are talking about the amount of pressure that oxygen exerts in arterial blood. This pressure is altered by certain changes within the body, including alveolar ventilation, barriers to gas exchange, temperature and pH.

If you imagine a lemonade bottle, the gas (in the case of lemonade, carbon dioxide) exerts a pressure in that solution – hence the fizz! If you shake the

Table 13.3 Normal ranges in arterial blood gas analysis.

pH	7.35–7.45
PaO_2	10–13 kPa
$PaCO_2$	4.5–6 kPa
HCO_3	17–23 mmol/l
BE	±2
SaO_2	95%

lemonade bottle the pressure exerted by the gas alters (i.e. it increases) and the lemonade fizzes over the top. At this point the analogy no longer works, as our patients do not fizz over and we don't shake them. However, the other factors listed above alter the partial pressure of oxygen in the same way as shaking the lemonade bottle alters the pressure exerted by the carbon dioxide within it.

Partial pressure of carbon dioxide – as above, but don't get confused with the lemonade bottle! Carbon dioxide is (indirectly) an acid, and in the presence of an enzyme called carbonic anhydrase (CA) it produces hydrogen ions. Therefore increasing concentrations of carbon dioxide lower the pH, making the blood become more acidic.

$$CO_2 + H_2O \overset{CA}{\leftrightarrow} H_2CO_3 \leftrightarrow H^+ + HCO_3^-$$

Hydrogen bicarbonate – this is the body's alkaline part of the balance (where carbon dioxide was the acid side). In general terms there should be 20 bicarbonate ions to every one carbon dioxide. If the pH of the body becomes too acidic (pH < 7.35) then the kidneys will retain more bicarbonate ions to maintain this ratio.

Base excess – this is also related to the alkaline control of the body and is a measure of the amount of available alkali/base. It is directly linked to hydrogen bicarbonate concentration. The more negative the base excess the more alkali has been utilised, i.e. the patient will be acidotic and hydrogen bicarbonate ions have been 'used up' to correct this. Therefore, there is very little excess base (alkali), so the base excess will be negative. The reverse is also true if the patient is alkalotic.

To interpret arterial blood gases you need to know the normal range for all the above parameters. Then use the guidelines in Figure 13.1. If you follow this simple method it will become easier to make sense of what you see. Causes of acidosis and alkalosis are shown in Table 13.4.

When the pH is abnormal for a while the body makes adjustments within the respiratory system and the renal system to either adjust the $PaCO_2$ levels or the amount of hydrogen bicarbonate ions excreted by the kidneys. This is called 'compensation'. The respiratory system can respond rapidly to facilitate respiratory compensation of a metabolic disturbance, but the renal system has a much slower response time (2–3 days).

A final note concerning blood gases is the definition of Type I and Type II respiratory failure.

Type I respiratory failure is the presence of hypoxia (PaO_2 < 10 kPa) but with *no* hypercapnia (i.e. a normal pCO_2).

Type II respiratory failure is the presence of hypoxia (PaO_2 < 10 kPa) *and* hypercapnia (pCO_2 > 6 kPa).

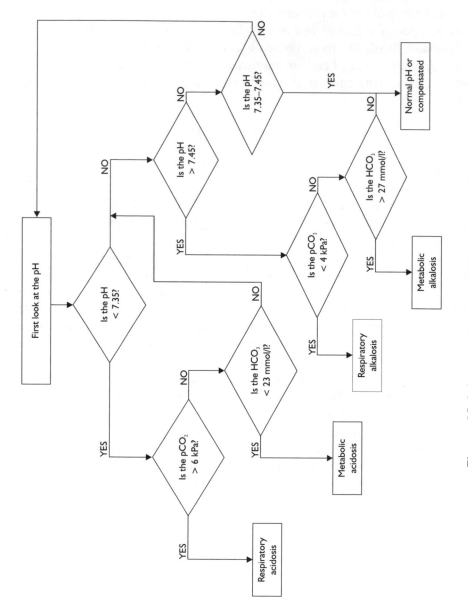

Figure 13.1 Interpreting arterial blood gas readings.

Table 13.4 Causes of acidosis/alkalosis.

Respiratory acidosis	Any condition that causes alveolar hypoventilation, e.g. COPD, Life threatening asthma, obstruction
	Opiate overdose
	Cardiac arrest
	Neurological damage
	Poisoning
Respiratory alkalosis	Any condition that causes alveolar hyperventilation
	Anxiety/hysteria
	Physiological response to hypoxia, e.g. pulmonary embolus, asthma
Metabolic acidosis	Diabetic ketoacidosis
	Lacticacidosis
	Renal tubular acidosis
	Septicaemia
	Ingestion of acid
Metabolic alkalosis	Prolonged vomiting
	Diarrhoea
	Gastric aspiration

Key point

Alkalosis is more dangerous than acidosis and more difficult to correct. You cannot inject a patient with acid to correct a metabolic alkalosis.

This chapter is a brief summary of the main components of respiratory assessment. Other assessment tools, such as peak flow and spirometry, are discussed in Chapter 9.

References

Turner, L. (2003) Pulse oximetry has its place but don't forget respiratory rate. *Nursing Times*, **98**, 40–65.

British Thoracic Society (2004) *Guidelines on Asthma.* `http://www.enterprise-portal2.co.uk/filestore/bts/asthmafull.pdf`.

Breakhall, A. (2004) The Respi-check oxygen mask. *British Journal of Resuscitation*, **3**(2), 21.

Carberry, M. (2002) Implementing the modified early warning system. *Nursing in Critical Care*, **7**(5), 220–6.

West, J. B. (2000) *Respiratory Physiology – The Essentials*, 6th edn. Lippincott Williams & Wilkins, Philadelphia.

Further reading

Scanlan, C. L., Wilkins, R. L. and Stoller, J. K. (1999) *Egan's Fundamentals of Respiratory Care*, 7th edn. Mosby, Missouri.

West, J. B. (1998) *Pulmonary Pathophysiology – The Essentials*, 5th edition. Lippincott Williams & Wilkins, Philadelphia.

CHAPTER 14

Respiratory failure and non-invasive positive pressure ventilation

Theresa Harvey

Respiratory failure is a complex subject to discuss. However, by understanding several simple principles it is much easier to address than you think. It can be acute, sub-acute, acute-on-chronic or chronic, and is dependant upon the stage of disease.

There are many definitions of respiratory failure, two of the better ones being:

> Respiratory failure is said to occur when the lung fails to oxygenate the arterial blood adequately and/or fails to prevent CO_2 retention. (West, 2000)

and

> Acute respiratory failure is a condition in which a stable $PaCO_2$, either normal or chronically increased cannot be maintained without extreme dyspnoea or mechanical support. (Rochester *et al.*, 1991)

Both of these statements reflect the comprehensive processes involved in respiratory failure. In order to understand this fully you need to recognise that there are two types of respiratory failure and that these are made up of four different mechanisms. These four mechanisms are known as hypoventilation, diffusion impairment, shunt and ventilation/perfusion (VQ) inequality (West, 2000). All four of these can be involved at one time, but the extent to which they influence respiratory failure can somewhat differ. It is important to appreciate that these mechanisms are important theoretical concepts and your ability to understand the processes involved will allow you to grasp why certain respiratory adjuncts (such as CPAP, NIV and oxygen therapy) are required when treating patients with failure.

The two types of respiratory failure are hypoxaemia and hypercapnia (West, 2000) and they can be termed hypoxaemic respiratory failure and hypercapnic respiratory failure (otherwise known as type I and type II respiratory failure respectively). The physiological and patho-physiological processes involved in both types of respiratory failure have similar principles, but can vary between patient groups.

Hypoxaemic respiratory failure

Hypoxaemic respiratory failure is related to a fall in the partial pressure of arterial and alveolar oxygen levels (PaO_2 and P_AO_2 respectively). Any four mechanisms can contribute to hypoxaemia and consequently to severe respiratory failure; however, the extent of the severity depends upon the pathology responsible for the hypoxaemia.

When *hypoventilation* is a cause of hypoxaemia there is a decrease in alveolar ventilation. Many of the factors influencing hypoventilation are thought to be extra-pulmonary in nature, such as trauma and neuromuscular dysfunction (Bach, 2002; West, 2000). Because hypoventilation is influenced by biomechanical elements it is not surprising to find that it is related to a failure in ventilation. As such, hypoventilation in hypoxaemia always coexists with hypercapnia. Of course, it should always be remembered that hypoventilation can be caused by respiratory depression and may sometimes be a result of biochemical changes.

A point to discuss before progressing is that when hypoxaemia presents secondary to hypoventilation, but alongside hypercapnia, it can be corrected relatively simply by the modest application of oxygen therapy (West, 2000). It may also be managed by the application of Positive End Expiratory Pressure (PEEP) in the form of Continuous Positive Airway Pressure (CPAP). This type of respiratory support is useful when high concentrations of oxygen are required (Mehta and Hill, 1996). Its application can splint the airways by raising Functional Residual Capacity (FRC), allowing lower concentrations of oxygen to be administered. Administering the lowest possible level of oxygen is very important when trying to avoid toxicity of the lung, a problem associated with sustained levels of high concentrations of oxygen (West, 2000).

Even though there may be an improvement and even a return to normal PaO_2 levels, there is a possibility that $PaCO_2$ will remain high, resulting in respiratory acidosis. Further issues of hypoventilation will be discussed later with hypercapnic respiratory failure (page 166).

Diffusion impairment can be seen in patients diagnosed with interstitial diseases, pneumonia(s) and pulmonary oedema, and is more frequently associated with exercise. This occurs due to an increased thickening of the alveolar–capillary membrane, which results in an inadequate equilibrium between gas and blood interfaces (West, 2000). This form of acute hypoxaemia is managed easily by the application of 100% oxygen (West, 2000), resulting in an increased P_AO_2 and overcoming any presenting hypoxaemia.

Shunts resulting in hypoxaemia can be extra-pulmonary and intra-pulmonary in nature. Shunt is the process that occurs when a portion of blood reaches the arterial circulation without passing a ventilated area of the lung (West, 2000) and can happen during Pulmonary Embolus (PE), severe lobular pneumonia and Acute Respiratory Distress Syndrome (ARDS). On their own, shunts have little or no influence on $PaCO_2$ and their management is not so easily treated by the use of 100% oxygen therapy. Depending upon the cause and extent of the hypoxaemia, overall acute management varies.

The major mechanism involved in all respiratory failure is *VQ inequality*. This is where various regions of the lung are ventilated but not matched by adequate blood flow. West (1998) describes this mechanism as 'the most common cause of hypoxaemia'. Here the normal pattern of VQ mismatching becomes disorganised, and can at times result in chronic hypoxaemia, which with acute illness becomes severely exaggerated.

A further consequence of VQ inequality is its influence on $PaCO_2$. This can become a problem if there is a change in respiratory drive, as is frequently seen in patients presenting with acute-on-chronic exacerbations of COPD. This discussion enters the realms of hypercapnic respiratory failure, which will be discussed later.

Some VQ inequalities can result in hypoxaemia alone, as seen in some emphysematous patients. Management here is around disease management, infection and appropriate oxygenation.

It is possible for these four mechanisms to coexist in acute respiratory failure. In order to avoid confusion there are several methods available that allow thorough investigation and accurate diagnosis/management. Such methods involve A–a gradient and Henderson–Hasselbalch equations. Both are complex in nature, but are very important in the assessment of respiratory failure. These techniques will not be discussed further, but can be found in any good respiratory physiology text. The more important *Gold Standard* measure to look out for is arterial blood gas analysis (ABG), and this is covered in Chapter 9.

Continuous Positive Airway Pressure in the management of acute hypoxaemic respiratory failure

Historically, hypoxaemic respiratory failure has been and is still managed by CPAP, and it is well documented to assist in the reversal of hypoxaemia

(Dehaven *et al.*, 1985; Gherini *et al.*, 1979; Lin *et al.*, 1995). More recently the use of non-invasive positive pressure ventilation (NIPPV) has been explored as an alternative option to CPAP, but the results have proved insignificant and there is little evidence to support its use in hypoxaemic respiratory failure.

CPAP is a widely used treatment and can be delivered in a variety of settings by a variety of professionals who are trained in its use. It is invaluable in the treatment of hypoxaemia and has been shown to reduce the incidence of intubation.

CPAP is the application of a continuous positive pressure that facilitates the 'splinting' of the airways throughout inspiration and expiration. It does so by raising the FRC using a measurement known as PEEP. This is attained by placing a predetermined valve onto the end of a high-flow system and by adding a specific mask to the system that the patient breathes through (Figure 14.1).

The overall physiological effects of CPAP are (Figures 14.2 and 14.3):

■ Increased FRC – pneumatic splinting of the airways
■ Mobilisation of secretions
■ Improved cardiovascular and pulmonary function (in pulmonary oedema)

Secondary benefits of raising FRC involve improvements on pulmonary compliance, with a decrease in the work/cost of breathing. It is also a treatment of choice for atelectasis (Gherini *et al.*, 1979) that may be due to both pathology and/or surgery. When CPAP is used to reverse atelectasis, it may well be used alongside physiotherapy techniques and manual hyperinflation (MHI).

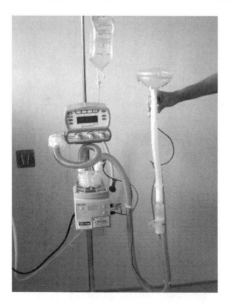

Figure 14.1 The Whisperflow CPAP system with humidification.

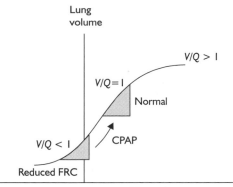

Figure 14.2 Effects of CPAP on FRC (copied with permission from Webber and Pryor, 1993).

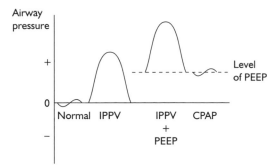

Figure 14.3 Positive pressure changes on FRC (copied with permission from Webber and Pryor, 1993).

MHI is vital to treat areas of collapse, but requires pressures of approximately 40 cm H_2O (Webber and Pryor, 1993), a pressure unobtainable by non-invasive CPAP alone. All of the above physiological effects result in an overall improvement in oxygenation and a rectification of presenting hypoxaemia which is usually due to a correction of ventilation–perfusion mismatching.

There are relative contraindications to CPAP and the following need consideration:

- Hypoventilation (risk of hypercapnia)
- Hypotension (systolic < 90)
- Unstable CVS and acute MI
- Reduced consciousness

- Undrained pneumothorax
- Head/face trauma
- Acute bronchospasm
- Broncho-pulmonary fistula
- Patient refusal or poor compliance

CPAP may also cause some complications. High intra-thoracic pressures may decrease cardiac output by affecting the ejection fraction from the ventricles, causing hypotension. There may be risk of aspiration secondary to gastric distension, vomiting and the continuous seal of the face mask. If the treatment is in place for any substantial duration of time there are also risks of dehydration and poor nutritional intake, along with the risk of pressure sores at the nasal bridge and chin.

If basic and routine care is in place these possible complications can be avoided by:

- Regular blood pressure observations within the first half an hour of application.
- Regular removal of face mask every hour to ensure hydration, coughing and pressure care.
- Possible insertion of a naso-gastric tube.
- Regular tracheostomy care when being delivered via a tracheostomy.
- Regular bronchodilator therapy if asthmatic.
- A regular check to any chest drains *in situ*.

If these simple steps can be taken it can greatly improve the safely and efficiency of the treatment CPAP.

Hypercapnic respiratory failure

Hypoventilation and VQ inequality are the two mechanisms involved in hypercapnic respiratory failure. In addition to these, the theoretical basis of load versus capacity (Rossi *et al.*, 1992) and the selective topic of respiratory muscle dysfunction are of great importance, especially when considering the role of NIV.

Hypoventilation and VQ inequality

Both of these mechanisms can be involved in hypercapnic respiratory failure. We have already discussed some issues around both hypoventilation and VQ inequality; however, there are key points to add which are specific to hypercapnia.

As discussed in hypoventilation, hypercapnia always coexists with hypoxaemia. The main point to consider in relation to hypercapnia is that its existence is secondary to poor alveolar ventilation, and as such its management lies with increasing ventilation. However, it is the role of VQ mismatch and its involvement in CO_2 retention that causes most debate. This occurs in acute chronic disease and the mismatch itself is secondary to disease process. There is a shift from normal values by disease process that leads to hypoxaemia and hypercapnia. In acute disease the sensitive chemoreceptors distributed around the body respond to these changes by increasing alveolar ventilation. This in turn reverses any hypercapnia to normal limits. However, in chronic disease the chemoreceptors may be unable to activate this physiological effect, leading to chronic hypercapnic respiratory failure. Reasons for this may lie in increased airway resistance and high respiratory loads/work of breathing (West, 1998).

Load versus capacity

Many patients (especially those with COPD) have increased expiratory and inspiratory loads on the respiratory muscles. These loads are influenced by factors that can increase load and decrease capacity (Keilty and Moxham, 1995). Initial reasoning for this increase in load lies with airways resistance caused by oedema, bronchospasm and secretions (see Figure 14.4). Because of gradual increases in resistance over a period of time, expiration becomes prolonged, resulting in increased lung emptying time.

In patients with COPD, this change over time results in dynamic hyperinflation, which in turn leads to the inability to reach functional residual capacity (FRC) before inspiration commences. This mechanism results in a physiological phenomenon known as intrinsic positive end expiratory pressure ($PEEP_i$) (Wedzicha, 1996) or gas trapping, as it is otherwise known. This form of PEEP splints open the floppy airways associated with COPD attempting to avoid atelectasis and airway closure. Unfortunately, this mechanism, when accompanied by the inability to empty the lungs compounds the problem of hyperinflation and places the respiratory muscles at a greater mechanical disadvantage.

When related to the pressure/volume curve, the tidal volume (V_T) is placed at a steeper transition of the curve. This compounds the problem even further by the additional work required to overcome $PEEP_i$. Such patients present with excessive accessory muscle use, a rapid shallow breathing pattern and altered chest shape, which on chest radiograph demonstrates flattened diaphragms (due to decreased zones of apposition), horizontal rib placement and elevated clavicles. Not only does working at this increased FRC impair capacity, but

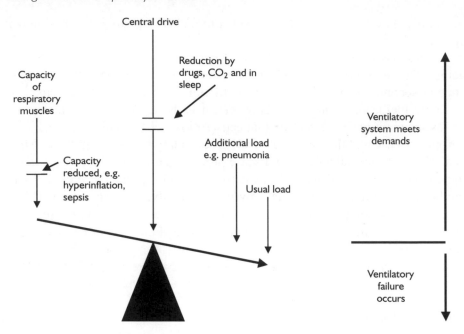

Figure 14.4 Load versus capacity in respiratory failure (Copied with permission from Kielty and Moxham, 1995).

it also results in a decrease in the muscle fibre length of the diaphragm and intercostals (Laghi, 2003).

Oedema, secretions and airway hyper-reactivity in the form of bronchospasm usually accompany exacerbations of COPD. If compounded by infection and copious secretion production, $PEEP_i$ may well increase, placing the respiratory pump under further stress. When such an acute exacerbation occurs the respiratory muscle pump becomes unbalanced, resulting in respiratory failure (Figure 14.4).

Respiratory muscle dysfunction

The above increases in load are related to a decreased capacity and mechanically disadvantaged muscles that may be compounded by fatigue (Polkey and Moxham, 1995), steroid induced weakness, malnutrition (Breslin, 1996) and worsening hypoxia and hypercapnia. Work by Juan *et al.* (1985) suggests that acidosis itself will restrict the contractile ability of the respiratory muscles, especially the diaphragm, placing further stresses upon the respiratory pump, precipitating the possible need for intubation.

Respiratory dysfunction is progressive and non-remitting. The consequence of respiratory muscle dysfunction is a decrease in respiratory muscle contractibility. This dysfunction can be bought about by a combination of weakness and fatigue. Both of these components lead to a decrease in the expected muscle force required to produce an adequate contraction for inspiration.

It is important to relate respiratory muscle dysfunction to respiratory failure; in fact it is due to chronic and acute-on-chronic dysfunction and the imbalances of load versus capacity occur. All elements related to respiratory failure and respiratory muscle dysfunction result in a profound effect on a patient's functional state and quality of life (Breslin, 1996), and these issues should always be addressed with dealing with both acute and chronic presentation.

Bi-level Positive Airway Pressure in the management of acute and acute-on-chronic hypercapnic respiratory failure

Many patients admitted to hospital with COPD present with uncompensated respiratory acidosis incorporating raised $PaCO_2$ levels and possible hypoxaemia. The management of such patients can be established by conservative means using steroid therapy, bronchodilators, antibiotics, oxygen therapy (Meduri, 1997; British Thoracic Society, 1997; Janssens *et al.*, 2000) and respiratory stimulants such as Doxapram (Jeffrey *et al.*, 1992; Moser *et al.*, 1973).

In the past, failure of such interventions to reverse the effects of respiratory acidosis would have inevitably resulted in the application of mechanical ventilation (Meduri, 1997; McGowan, 1998; Kaminski and Kaplan, 1999). The complications associated with endotracheal intubation (nosocomial pneumonia, laryngeal and tracheal injury, impaired haemodynamics) and ventilation have been well documented (Brochard, 1996; Ho and Boyle, 2000). In addition to these common complications, others, such as sinusitis, sepsis and decreased cardiac output, have been seen (Ambrosino, 1996). The consequence of mechanically ventilating patients with COPD results in significant morbidity and mortality (Moore and Schmidt, 2001), with a documented mortality rate of 12–19% (Ambrosino, 1996), and this is not to mention any difficulties encountered when attempting to wean surviving patients (Brochard, 1996). NIV has since been shown to reduce the need for intubation, avoiding such complications, and as such has had a resurgence of popularity throughout the world.

It is important to consider that the majority of hypercapnic patients coming to the admissions unit or emergency room may be COPD patients. However, there are other patient groups presenting with this pattern of respiratory failure,

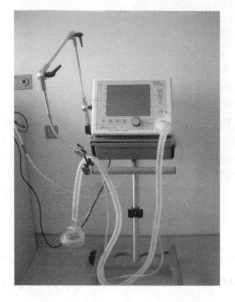

Figure 14.5 The BiPAP Vision (Respironics).

such as those with neurological disease and suppressed central drive (opoid abuse or over-sedation). It is also important to remember that many patients who develop hypercapnic respiratory failure may already be existing inpatients who may be exhausting or returning from theatre.

There are a variety of machines (Figures 14.5 and 14.6) and interfaces (face and nasal) available for use in non-invasive ventilation and its application occurs throughout both acute (including A&E/wards/HDUs and ITUs) and domiciliary settings, and it is initiated and managed by a multitude of specialist professionals. There are two types of machine, controlled by either pressure or volume. There is little evidence to suggest that one mode is more effective than another; however, pressure-controlled machines are used more widely than those controlled by volume as an emergency adjunct in acute respiratory failure.

There is debate as to when BiPAP should be initiated and how it should be managed. The BTS guidelines on NIV outline many of these issues. It should be initiated alongside a thorough medical regime, and a plan including resuscitation state and ITU admission status should be clearly documented. There should be a strict protocol in place for the management of BiPAP, including frequency of ABGs, titration, rest periods and observations.

BiPAP runs along similar principles to CPAP in that the same contraindications and complications apply. It is in the indications for use that CPAP and NIV differ, and the BTS Guidelines (Baudouin *et al.*, 2002) suggest its use in/when:

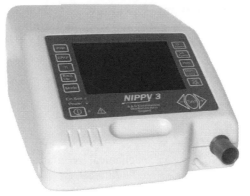

Figure 14.6 The NiPPY 3 (B&D Electromedical).

- pH = 7.25–7.35
- Patients weaning from mechanical ventilation
- Hypercapnia secondary to chest wall deformity or neuro-muscular disease
- Cardiogenic pulmonary oedema not responding to CPAP

NIV uses two pressures known as IPAP (Inspiratory Positive Airway Pressure) and EPAP (Expiratory Positive Airway Pressure). The EPAP performs in exactly the same way that CPAP does, in that it improves oxygenation by raising the FRC. However, the key difference is in the IPAP. This higher pressure influences the movement of gases throughout the respiratory cycle and facilitates adequate tidal volumes, facilitating the movement of CO_2 out of the pulmonary system. Figure 14.3 shows how this mode of ventilation (referred to as IPPV) augments FRC and tidal volumes especially when compared to CPAP.

Another key feature in any NIV is the use of respiratory rate backup facilities. Here a pre-set rate of usually 8–12 is adjusted as part of the machine setup. This ensures adequate ventilation of the patient should apnoea occur. This is important in hypercapnic respiratory failure due to CO_2 narcosis and suppressed respiratory drive. Despite having this backup facility it should be stressed that BiPAP should only be initiated on spontaneously breathing patients who are able to trigger the machine independently. Any patients with a fluctuating GCS should be considered for more invasive management.

Once commenced, BiPAP should be monitored closely for the first 1–2 hours with regard to arterial blood gas analysis and routine observations. By this stage there should be signs of improvement. Progression involves stabilising the patient and normalising blood gases to the patient's normal parameters. Once this has been attained, BiPAP can be used intermittently (especially at night) until the patient is able to manage off the machine.

If there are no signs of improvement after 1–2 hours it may be prudent to inform intensive care outreach teams and seek their opinion, as NIV failure can delay intubation and have an impact upon mortality.

References

Ambrosino, N. (1996). Noninvasive mechanical ventilation in acute respiratory failure. *European Respiratory Journal*, **9**, 795–807.

Bach, J. R. (2002) *Non-invasive Mechanical Ventilation*. Hanley & Belfus, Philadelphia.

Baudouin, S., Blumenthal, S., Cooper, B., Davidson, C., Davison, A., Elliott, A., Kinnear, W., Patron, R., Sawicka, E. and Turner, L. (2002) Noninvasive ventilation in acute respiratory failure. *Thorax*, **57**, 192–211.

Breslin, E. H. (1996) Respiratory muscle function in patients with chronic obstructive pulmonary disease. *Heart and Lung*, **25**(4), 271–87.

Brochard, L. (1996). Non-invasive ventilation in acute respiratory failure. *Respiratory Care*, **41**(5), 456–65.

Brochard, L., Mancebo, J., Wysocki, M., Lofaso, F., Conti, G., Rauss, A., Simonneau, G., Benito, S., Gasparetto, A., Lemaire, F., Isabey, D. and Harf, A. (1995). Non-invasive positive pressure ventilation for acute exacerbations of chronic obstructive pulmonary disease. *New England Journal of Medicine*, **333**(13), 817–22.

British Thoracic Society (BTS) (1997) Guidelines on the management of COPD. *Thorax* , **52**(suppl V).

Dehaven, C. B., Hurst, J. M. and Branson, R. D. (1985) Post extubation hypoxaemia treated with continuous positive airways pressure mask. *Critical Care Medicine*, **13**(1), 46–8.

Gherini, S., Peters, R. M. and Virglio, R. M. (1979). Mechanical work of breathing with positive end expiratory pressure and continuous positive airways pressure. *Chest*, **76**, 251–6.

Ho, R. P. Y. and Boyle, M. (2000) Non-invasive positive pressure ventilation in acute respiratory failure: providing competent care. *Australian Critical Care*, **13**(4), 143.

Janssens, J.-P., De Muralt, B. and Titelion, V. (2000) Management of dyspnoea in severe chronic obstructive pulmonary disease. *Journal of Pain and Symptom Management*, **19**(5), 378–92.

Jeffrey, A. A., Warren, P. M. and Flenley, D. C. (1992). Acute hypercapnic respiratory failure in patients with chronic obstructive lung disease: risk factors and use of guidelines for management. *Thorax*, **47**, 34–40.

Juan, G., Calverey, P., Talamo, C., Schnader, J. and Roussos, C. (1985) Effect of carbon dioxide on diaphragmatic function in human beings. *New England Journal of Medicine*, **310**, 874–9.

Kaminski, J. and Kaplan, P. D. (1999) The role of noninvasive positive pressure ventilation in the emergency department. *Topics in Emergency Medicine*, **21**(4), 68–73.

Keilty, S. E. J. and Moxham, J. (1995) Noninvasive ventilation in acute-on-chronic airways disease. *Hospital Update*, April.

Laghi, F. and Tobin, M. J. (2001). Disorders of the respiratory muscles. *American Journal of Respiratory Critical Care Medicine*, **168**(1), 10–48.

Lin, M. (1995) Reappraisal of continuous positive airways pressure therapy in acute cardiogenic pulmonary oedema: short-term results and long term follow-up. *Chest*, **107**(5), 1370–86.

McGowan, C. M. (1998) Non-invasive ventilatory support: use of bi-level positive airway pressure in respiratory failure. *Critical Care Nurse*, **18**(6), 47–53.

Meduri, G. U. (1997) Noninvasive positive pressure ventilation in chronic obstructive pulmonary disease patients with acute exacerbation. *Critical Care Medicine*, **25**(10), 1631–3.

Mehta, S. and Hill, N. S. (1996) Non-invasive ventilation in acute respiratory failure. *Respiratory Care Clinics of North America*, **2**, 267–92.

Moore, M. J. and Schmidt, G. A. (2001) Keys to effective non-invasive ventilation, Part 1: Initial steps. *Journal of Critical Illness*, **16**(2), 64–70.

Moser, K. M., Luchsinger, P. C., Adamson, J. S., McMahon, S. M., Schlueter, D. P., Spivack, M. and Weg, J. G. (1973) Respiratory stimulation with intravenous doxapram in respiratory failure. A double-blind co-operative study. *New England Journal of Medicine*, **228**(9), 427–31.

Plant, P. K., Owen, J. L. and Elliott, M. W. (2000) Early use of non-invasive ventilation for acute exacerbations of chronic obstructive pulmonary disease on general respiratory wards: a multicentre randomised controlled trial. *The Lancet*, **355**, 1931–5.

Polkey, M. I. and Moxham, J. (1995) Non-invasive ventilation in the management of decompensated COPD. *Monaldi Archives of Chest Disease*, **50**(5), 378–82.

Rochester, D. F. (1991) The diaphragm in COPD. Better than expected but not good enough. *New England Journal of Medicine*, **325**(13), 917–23.

Rossi, A., Polese, G. and De Sandre, G. (1992) Respiratory failure in chronic airflow obstruction: recent advances and therapeutic implications in the critically ill patient. *European Journal on Medicine*, **1**(6), 349–57.

Webber, B. A. and Pryor, J. J. (1993) *Physiotherapy for Respiratory and Cardiac Problems*. Churchill Livingstone, London.

Wedzicha, J. A. (1996) Non-invasive ventilation for exacerbations of respiratory failure in chronic obstructive pulmonary disease. *Thorax*, **52**(Suppl 2), S35–S39.

West, J. B. (1998) *Pulmonary Pathophysiology: The Essentials*, 5th edn. Lippincott Williams & Wilkins, London.

West, J. B. (2000) *Respiratory Physiology: The Essentials*. 6th edn. Lippincott Williams & Wilkins, London.

CHAPTER 15

Smoking cessation

Sarah Lea

Introduction

Adult smoking prevalence in the UK over the past 20 years has fallen (Department of Health, 2000a), but despite this in 2000 about 12.5 million adults in the UK smoked cigarettes – 29% of men and 25% of women – and women's rates are catching up, particularly in new smokers (Royal College of Nursing, 2001a). The addictiveness of smoking and the health risks involved are well documented: cigarettes have an addictive pull estimated to be over 10 times more powerful than heroin (Royal College of Physicians, 2000).

The increasing cost of health care associated with an ageing population and chronic disease patterns makes smoking reduction a priority in trying to reduce the burden by improving people's health and health outcomes.

The Government has put resources and funding in place to try to reduce smoking prevalence, by means of health education and smoking cessation services, by 21% by 2010 (Department of Health, 1998a). The majority of smokers admit that it is harmful, and it is estimated that one in three want to stop. Over half of smokers will eventually be killed by their habit (Department of Health, 1998b). Around 300 smokers die per day (Croghan, 2005), and it causes chronic ill health in many more.

The physiological effects of smoking

Smoking damages the respiratory system, but while some people notice the more obvious side-effects of smoking, they do not appreciate its effect on their lung function (Shuttleworth, 2004).

Lung disease associated with smoking has a gradual onset of chronic cough, winter infections and breathlessness on exertion (Milner, 2004). People often put their symptoms down to the ageing process or they go unnoticed until they become severe enough for them to seek medical advice. The stigma of smoking can also delay presenting for help. The most common respiratory diseases caused by smoking are Chronic Obstructive Pulmonary Disease (COPD) and lung cancer. A study of male British doctors for forty years showed that smoking caused 81% of lung cancer deaths and 78% of deaths with COPD (Doll *et al.*, 1994). This led to a rapid decline in smoking rates amongst doctors, not mirrored within other health care professionals. Smoking causes a more rapid decline in lung function than naturally occurs within the ageing process (Fletcher and Peto, 1977). Smoking cessation should be the first form of therapy offered to people with mild airways disease (Anthonisen *et al.*, 1994). It is also responsible for fatal diseases in other parts of the body: it is the prime cause of other cancers, heart disease and stroke. It can exacerbate other chronic diseases and fatal conditions.

To understand how lung disease is caused by smoking you need to identify the toxic components in tobacco smoke.

The ASH web site (`http://www.ash.org.uk/`) lists over 4,000 chemicals contained in tobacco leaves. ASH also lists the known human carcinogens found in cigarette smoke; it is these, rather than nicotine, that cause cancer. Smoking is described as having a gas and particulate phase. Cigarettes also contain additives which may increase the nicotine in the gas phase and cause increased absorption.

Box 15.1 The effects of smoking on health

Smoking causes:

- 84% of deaths from lung cancer
- 83% of deaths from COPD
- 30% of cancer deaths in addition to lung cancer: cancer of mouth, larynx, oesophagus, bladder, kidney, stomach and pancreas
- 14% of deaths from heart disease

Smoking is also linked to other serious conditions, including:

- Asthma
- Osteoporosis

Box 15.2 Carcinogens in human cigarettes

- Aromatic amines (2-naphthylamines and 4-aminobiphenyl)
- Benzene
- Vinyl chloride
- Ethylene chloride
- Arsenic
- Nickel
- Chromium
- Cadmium
- Radioactive element (polonium-210)
- Possible significant human carcinogens: benzo(a)pyrene, nitros-amines, aldehydes, acrylonitrile, DDT, cobalt and lead

Box 15.3 Constituents of the gas phase of cigarette smoking

- Acetone
- Acrolein (this damages the hair-like cilia in the upper airways causing particulate matter to collect in the airways and lungs)
- Ammonia (an irritant of the airways)
- Carbon monoxide (reduces the blood's oxygen-carrying capacity and inhibits respiration)
- Carbon dioxide
- Nitrogen
- Hydrogen
- Methane
- Nitrogen oxides (cause lung inflammation)
- Polycyclic aromatic hydrocarbons
- Phenol
- Hydrogen sulphide
- Hydrogen cyanide
- Volatile nitriles
- Toluene
- Formaldehyde
- Benzene

Nicotine is found in the particulate phase of smoking. It increases in the gas phase as the pH of the smoke becomes alkaline.

Clinical damage

Damage is caused to the lungs in three main ways:

- Mucus hypersecretion
- Alveolar destruction
- Inflammatory changes in the airways

Increased mucus secretion and inflammation cause obstruction of peripheral airways. The airways are normally held open by alveolar attachments, but in smoking-related airways damage these are reduced, leading to airways closure (Barnes, 1999).

Smoking-related issues

The decline in lung function and its acceleration by smoking was identified by Fletcher and Peto in 1977 (Figure 15.1).

It is known that many people present with symptoms of smoking-related airways damage when they have lost 50% or more of their lung function, mainly between the ages of 50 and 70 (Bellamy and Booker, 2004). Viral colds and winter bronchitis can cause a sudden decline; post-infective symptoms which do not subside can mean frequent GP consultations; and further investigations and testing with spirometry can lead to the diagnosis of COPD.

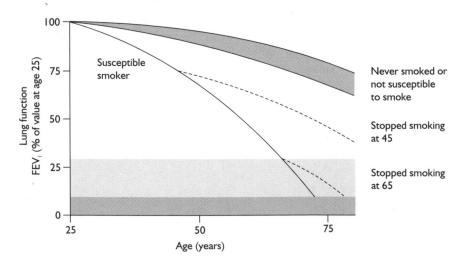

Figure 15.1 The decline in lung function, effects of smoking.

Although stopping smoking does not help people regain their lost lung function, it can help to slow its decline to that of a non-smoker (Fletcher and Peto, 1977).

Screening susceptible smokers is important in identifying at-risk people or those with early disease. Nurses in primary and secondary care are carrying out more nurse-led respiratory clinics with lung function testing.

The new GMS2 contract in primary care promotes lung function testing, with spirometry as part of the screening and ongoing care of respiratory patients and the recording of smoking status (Booker, 2004).

Educating people about the benefits of smoking cessation, offering advice and support, is an important part of this work. Recording smoking status gives an ideal opportunity for health promotion and a chance to impress on smokers that it is never too late to stop in order to benefit their health.

The nurse's role in helping people to quit

Nurses' knowledge varies greatly in their ability to provide smoking cessation advice. Many nurses have taken specialist training, either through their local stopping smoking service, or as part of a respiratory or nurse prescribing course, and run clinics as part of their wider role.

The Royal College of Nursing (2001a) recommends the use of the 5 As (below) as a quick intervention; a more detailed guide is available in Royal College of Nursing (2001b).

- **Ask**
All patients should be asked their smoking status as a routine question at an appropriate time. Such as on admission, pre-admission assessment, clinic or routine appointment.

- **Advise**
To quit is the single most important thing they can do to improve their health.

- **Assess**
Ask if they are ready to quit if they are provided with the information and resources and assistance to do it. Offer information about the health benefits of quitting and help patients to identify barriers to quitting. Give contact details of support services for the future.

- **Assist**
Encourage patients to set a quit date, ideally within two weeks. Develop a plan to include coping strategies, and enlisting help from friends and family.

■ **Arrange**

Refer those who want to quit to a smoking cessation service for specialist ongoing help and support.

Being able to give telephone numbers for local or national helplines should be the minimal intervention by the nurse. Hopefully, this will start thoughts about quitting and lead to the seeking of further advice, even if they are not able to quit at that time. People often ask if the nurse smokes, possibly to seek approval or to see if the nurse has an understanding of how difficult it is to quit. Nurses should try not to smoke in front of patients and should act as role models. NHS sites will hopefully become smoke-free zones in the near future.

Nurses who smoke should aim to give impartial advice. It has been proved that even brief intervention does have an effect in encouraging people to move forward in the quitting process (Milner, 2004).

Simple interventions by key workers, such as doctors, nurses and GPs, have been recognised as vital and effective in helping people to quit (Percival, 2005; Bellamy and Booker, 2004). Reinforcement can increase the quit rate from 10% to 30%, which equates to an extra 350,000 quitters per year (Silagy and Stead, 2002).

NRT and Bupropion: what's available?

The principle of NRT is to replace nicotine at a lower level than smoking, reducing withdrawal symptoms and allowing smokers to change their habit of smoking (Bellamy and Booker, 2004).

Nurses undergoing specialist prescriber training have been able to prescribe nicotine replacement therapy since the introduction of the Nurse Prescribers' Extended Formulary (NPEF) in April 2002 (Baird, 2006). This specialist training has allowed nurses to work more effectively in nurse-led clinics and to give access to help, support and prescriptions to people in their own homes.

Nurses build up relationships with people, and this has been said to help in promoting smoking cessation (Fendell and MacDonald, 2005). It is recognised that there are concerns about using NRT in certain groups of people, such as pregnant or breastfeeding women, or within three months of a heart attack or stroke (Bellamy and Booker, 2004; British National Formulary, 2005).

Concerns about doing harm to people with specific diseases can also mean the need to weigh up the pros and cons of treatment. In most cases opinions suggest that NRT is much safer than continuing to smoke (McNeill *et al.*, 2001). In complex cases further medical or pharmaceutical advice should always be sought, and all cautions and contraindications listed in the British National Formulary (2005) taken into account before making a prescribing decision. The use of NRT can double long-term quit rates (Bellamy and Booker, 2004).

National guidelines provided by National Institute for Clinical Excellence (2002) advise the NHS to fund a smoking cessation attempt every six months in people who commit to a stop date (British National Formulary, 2005) to encourage smokers to quit. NRT is made available on FP10 (an NHS prescription) and those eligible pay a prescription charge.

Being able to afford to use NRT is therefore not a real issue in a committed quitter – a 20 per day smoker would spend £31,025 over the next 20 years (http://www.ash.org.uk/). Easier access to NRT products over the counter (OTC) in pharmacies and supermarkets has increased the availability of products, and pharmacists can offer specialist advice and support to people wanting to quit.

If an interested smoker is not ready to quit then a later date could be set to discuss things again.

Certain factors should be taken into account when considering which therapy to give:

- Smoker's likely compliance
- Availability of counselling and support
- Previous experience of smoking cessation aids
- Contra-indications and adverse reactions of products
- Patient preferences (British National Formulary, 2005) .

Usually a prescription is given for two weeks' treatment. This allows for early follow-up support and to discuss any issues or problems with the therapy. The prescription length increases if the person shows commitment to quitting. Encouragement should always be given to take the full course of NRT, as trying to quit too soon has been shown to be more likely to fail (Percival, 2005; Bellamy and Booker, 2004). It is useful to discuss factors in the home and work environment which may need to change in order to succeed in quitting, such as telling people that you are stopping. Quit with a friend, get rid of ashtrays, ask other people not to smoke around you, do something else with your hands and change the daily routine to reduce opportunities to smoke. Nicotine replacement therapy is seen as the pharmacological treatment in managing smoking cessation in those smoking 10 cigarettes a day or more (British National Formulary, 2005).

Nicotine skin patch

- Available in either a 16 or 24 hour strength patch. Usually applied to clean dry skin in the morning.

- Available in three strengths with a 12 week quit programme. Most people start on the higher strength patch.
- Some people have problems with the adhesive, such as irritation or not sticking. They are available in two types: clear and pink/beige.
- In deciding which patch to offer the prescriber takes into account the amount and pattern of smoking.
- Advice should always be given on the potential side effects of treatment (British National Formulary, 2005) and the need for will-power and commitment to quitting. Some side-effects, if experienced, with the 24 hour patches can be reduced by changing to a 16 hour patch.

Nicotine nasal spray

- A solution of nicotine is squirted directly into the nostrils. It is absorbed fast and may suit heavy smokers.
- It can cause irritation of the nasal passages. The dose is reduced gradually over 12 weeks with a maximum of 12 weeks use.

Nicotine chewing gum

- Available in 2 mg or 4 mg doses in different flavours.
- One brand of this product is also licensed for 'cut down and quit' (see 'Cut down then stop' strategy on the ASH web site).
- It should be chewed slowly, which releases the nicotine into the side of the mouth, and then kept in the side of the mouth to release into the mucous membrane for about 30 minutes per piece.
- Treatment does not usually exceed six months. People using the cut down and quit approach should set a stop date for smoking. Nicotine swallowed is inactive. Most people use the 2 mg dose, as 4 mg is for very heavy smokers only.

Nicotine inhalator

- Consists of a plastic mouthpiece with nicotine cartridges that fit into the end of the device. Nicotine is absorbed in the mouth and throat and not into the lungs. Smokers draw on it like a cigarette. The cartridge lasts about 20 minutes.

- Abstinence should be achieved within three months. Also used in the 'cut down and stop' programme (ASH web site).

Micro tab

- Placed under the tongue it dissolves slowly, releasing 2 mg of nicotine. Suitable for smokers of 20 cigarettes or more daily. Used on demand the peak nicotine level is similar to that of the gum or inhalator (Bellamy and Booker, 2004). Programme of reduction should not usually exceed six months.

Lozenges

- Available in 2 mg and 4 mg doses, they are sucked to release nicotine through the mucous membrane of the mouth. One or two lozenges can be sucked per hour. They are sugar free, and the aim is to reduce the dose over 3 months with a maximum of 6 months' treatment.

Non-nicotine-based treatment: Bupropion (Zyban) and Champix (Varenicline)

This treatment has been shown to have a quit rate of up to 30% when used in conjunction with counselling and support, and can double long-term/one year smoking cessation rates (Bellamy and Booker, 2004). In tablet form it is used over a two-month period, but is not suitable for everyone. Bupropion is only available on prescription as it has some serious contraindications and side-effects (British National Formulary, 2005).

Before a prescribing decision is made a full medical and pharmacological history should be taken, including OTC and herbal therapies, to check suitability for this treatment (British National Formulary, 2005). Originally used as an antidepressant, it works by reducing the desire to smoke by sensitising the brain's nicotine receptors and reducing withdrawal symptoms (Jorenby *et al.*, 1999; Bellamy and Booker, 2004).

The smoker quits during the second week of treatment. It can also be used with an NRT patch and its use doubles the chance of quitting (Jorenby *et al.*, 1999).

Bupropion has been endorsed by the National Institute for Clinical Excellence (2002) because it has better quit rates than other methods and is cost-effective.

Champix is a relatively new medication available on prescription which is used to relieve the craving and withdrawal symptoms of stopping smoking and is also claimed to reduce the enjoyment of continuing to smoke. It is taken in tablet form and the dose is titrated upwards as the course continues. It may alter the efficacy of other medications, such as theophylline and warfarin, which may require an adjustment in dose. Common side-effects include headache, nausea, abnormal dreams and difficulty in sleeping.

Box 15.4 Withdrawal symptoms after stopping smoking

■ Cravings
Intense at first; last 2 to 3 minutes but become less frequent during the first three weeks.

■ Increased appetite
As nicotine has suppressed the appetite and increased metabolism, people can gain weight, but this can be minimal if they control their diet as their metabolism adjusts.

■ Anxiety, irritability and loss of concentration
Upheaval of breaking a long-term habit and adjusting to physical changes.

■ Sleep disturbance
Not uncommon. Initially unable to sleep, followed by a week of difficulty trying to stay awake.

■ Worsening cough
This happens as cilia in the respiratory tract start to function again. It is temporary.

■ Light-headedness or dizziness
Rarely lasts more than 2–3 days: carbon monoxide in the blood is being replaced by oxygen.

■ Throat or mouth ulcers
Caused by chemical and bacterial changes in the mouth.

■ Constipation
Tobacco has a laxative effect (Percival, 2005).

Outcomes of interventions

Despite all of the resources available, many people fail to quit, or relapse shortly after quitting. Very few smokers succeed at their first attempt (Youden *et al.*, 2005). Smokers who try to give up without help have a 1–3 per cent change of success (Fowler, 2004). NRT increases long-term quit rates by 1.5 to 2-fold. Follow-up and support are critical in the first 2–3 weeks (Bellamy and Booker, 2004).

Success rates with NRT and advice from a healthcare professional are increased and maximised with ongoing support and education (Wilson, 2000; Silagy and Stead, 2002).

Quitters need to be made aware of the withdrawal symptoms of smoking, as it is often these that start them smoking again.

NRT is cost-effective in helping people to stop smoking (British National Formulary, 2005). A list of the benefits of quitting can be used to allow an understanding of the process of recovery and to encourage sustained abstinence.

Benefits of quitting: time after last cigarette

- *20 minutes*: Blood pressure and pulse return to normal; circulation improves in hands and feet, making them warmer.
- *8 hours*: Oxygen levels in the blood return to normal; chances of a heart attack start to fall.
- *24 hours*: Carbon monoxide is eliminated from the body; mucus and other debris start to clear from the lungs.
- *48 hours*: Nicotine is no longer detected in the body; ability to taste and smell improves.
- *72 hours*: Breathing becomes easier as the bronchial tubes relax; energy levels increase.
- *2–12 weeks*: Circulation improves in the body, making walking easier.
- *3–9 months*: Breathing problems such as cough, shortness of breath and wheeze slowly improve; lung function increases by about 5–10%.
- *5 years*: Heart attack risk falls to about half that of a smoker.
- *10 years*: Risk of lung cancer falls to half that of a smoker. Risk of heart attack similar to never smoker; five-year risk of heart attack falls to about half of that of a smoker (Health Authority, 1994).

In conclusion, nurses should remember that although some people are able to stop on their own, it is important that they should be able to give up-to-date advice about the treatments and resources available to those who need it. Help-ing smokers to give up is one of the most cost effective health interventions, and nurses are in a unique position to fill that role (Youden *et al.*, 2005).

Smoking cessation work can be rewarding. Skills gained can be shared with colleagues to encourage formation of more clinics and services run by nurses. Local funding for training and development of skills is more read-ily available since the Government's initiatives to target smoking and reduce health inequality (Department of Health, 2000b).

Smokers expect health professionals to address their smoking, and health economists rate stopping smoking as a highly cost-effective use of NHS resources, saving the NHS the cost of treating other illness before it arises (World Health Organization, 2001).

In the UK, smoking cessation has proved excellent value for money, and absti-nence rates and long-term quit rates have been shown to be increased by NRT and intensive support, in equal division (Royal College of Nursing, 2001a).

References

Anthonisen, N. R., Connett, J. E., Kiley, J. P., Altose, M. D., Bailey, W. C., Buist, A. S., Conway, W. A. Jr, Enright, P. L., Kanner, R. E., O'Hara. P. *et al.* (1994). Effects of smoking intervention and the use of as inhaled anticholinergic broncholilator on the rate of decline of FEV1: the lung health study. *Journal of the American Medi-cal Association*, **272**, 1497–505.

Baird, A. (2006) Prescription for change. *RCN Magazine*, Spring, 21–5.

Barnes, P. (1999) *Managing Chronic Obstructive Pulmonary Disease*, pp. 8–10. Sci-ence Press, London.

Bellamy, D. and Booker, R. (2004) *Chronic Obstructive Pulmonary Disease in Pri-mary Care*, 3rd edn, pp. 13, 68–77. Class Publishing, London.

British National Formulary (2005) *British National Formulary* (ed. D. Mehta), pp. 260–2. British Medical Association and Royal Pharmaceutical Society of Great Britain, London.

Booker, R. (2004) The new GMS contract: COPD management and GMS. *Practice Nurse*, **27**(10), 20–8.

Coleman, T. and Wilson, A. (2000) Anti-smoking advice from General Practitioners: is a population-based approach to advice-giving feasible? *British Journal of General Practice*, **50**, 1001–4.

Croghan, E. (2005) Smoking related health risks are every nurse's business. *Nursing Times*, **101**(23), 16.

Department of Health (1998a) *Smoking Kills. A White Paper on Tobacco*. HMSO, London.

Department of Health (1998b) *The UK Smoking Epidemic: Deaths in 1995*. Health Education Authority, London.

Department of Health (2000a) *The NHS Plan. A Plan for Investment. A Plan for Reform.* http://www.nhsia.nhs.uk/nhsplan/.

Department of Health (2000b) Statistics on smoking, England, 1978 onwards. *Department of Health Statistics Bulletin.* Department of Health, London.

Doll, R., Peto, R., Wheatley, K., Gray, R. and Sutherland, I. (1994) Mortality in relation to smoking: 40 years observations on male British doctors. *British Medical Journal*, **309**, 901–11.

Fendell, L. and MacDonald, T. (2005) cited in Shuttleworth A. (2005) A key role in smoking cessation. *Nursing Times*, **701**(30), 22.

Fletcher, C. and Peto, R. (1977) The natural history of chronic airflow obstruction. *British Medical Journal*, **6077**, 1645–8.

Fowler, C. (2004) Smoking: time to confront a major health issue. Update (suppl), 6 May.

Health Authority (1994), p. 20. Adapted from Fletcher and Peto (1977); cited in Royal College of Nursing (2001) *Clearing the Air 2*, p. 20. Royal College of Nursing, London.

Jorenby, D. E., Leischow, S., Nides, M., Rennard, S., Johnston, J. A., Hughes, A. R., Smith, S. S., Muramoto, M. L., Daughton, D. M., Doan, K., Fiore, M. C. and Baker, T. B. (1999) A controlled trial of sustained-release Bupropion, a nicotine patch, or both for smoking cessation. *New England Journal of Medicine*, **340**, 685–91.

McNeill, A., Foulds, J. and Bates, C. (2001) Regulation of nicotine replacement therapies. A critique of current practice. *Addiction*, **96**(12), 1757–68.

Milner, D. (2004) The physiological effects of smoking on the respiratory system. *Nursing Times*, **100**(24), 56–9.

National Institute for Clinical Excellence (2002) *Guidance on the Use of Nicotine Replacement Therapy (NRT and Bupropion) for Smoking Cessation.* National Institute for Clinical Excellence, London. http//www.nice.org.uk/.

Percival, J. (2005) Helping people to stop smoking: the role of treatment products. *Nursing Times*, **101**(48), 52–4.

Royal College of Nursing (2001) *Clearing the Air 2: Smoking and Tobacco Control – an Updated Guide for Nurses.* Royal College of Nursing, London.

Royal College of Physicians (2000) *Nicotine Addiction in Britain. A Report of the Tobacco Advisory Groups of the Royal College of Physicians.* Royal College of Physicians, London.

Shuttleworth, A. (2004) The role of nurses in reducing the use of tobacco (Smoking cessation initiatives by non-specialist hospital nurse). *Nursing Times*, **100**(1), 24–5.

Silagy, C. and Stead, L. F. (2002) Physician advice for smoking cessation (Cochrane Review). *The Cochrane Library*, Issue 4.

World Health Organization (2001) *The Case for Commissioning Smoking Cessation Services.* WHO Europe Partnership Project and SmokeFree, London. Available from http://www.ash.org.uk/?cessation/.

CHAPTER 16

Tuberculosis

Helen Thuraisingham

Although often considered a disease of the past, tuberculosis (TB) continues to present a serious threat to public health in the UK. Worldwide it is estimated that it kills two million people every year and causes more deaths than any other single infectious disease (World Health Organization, 2005; Health Protection Agency, 2005). Countries with a high incidence of TB are those with more than 40 cases of TB per 100,000 population (World Health Organization, 2005). This means that all countries except those in Western Europe, North America, Canada, Australia and New Zealand have an increased risk from tuberculosis. In England and Wales there has continued to be an increase in the number of cases notified since 1993 (Health Protection Agency, 2005).

Tuberculosis is an infectious bacterial disease spread from one person to another mainly by airborne transmission. The causal organism is the tubercule bacillus *Mycobacterium tuberculosis* and variants such *Mycobacterium bovis*. Tuberculosis can affect any organ of the body; however, pulmonary tuberculosis is the most frequent site of involvement and it is usually only pulmonary TB that is infectious (Ait-Khaled and Enarson, 2003).

Tuberculosis causes two main states: tuberculosis infection (latent TB) and tuberculosis disease (active TB). With latent TB infection, mycobacteria are present in the body but remain dormant, with the potential to activate or reactivate disease. Tuberculosis disease is present when the bacilli are actively dividing and symptoms develop. It has been demonstrated that about 30% of healthy individuals closely exposed to TB will become infected. Of those, 5–10% will go on to develop active disease (Health Protection Agency, 2005).

Point for thought

Consider how world travel has changed over the last 20 years. What impact do you think this may have on the global distribution of tuberculosis?

When people with pulmonary tuberculosis speak, cough or sneeze, they produce an aerosol of droplets from the bronchial tree that contains tubercule bacilli; these droplets have the potential to be infectious. Two essential factors determine the risk of transmission to a healthy person: the concentration of the infected droplets suspended in the air, and the period of time during which the exposed individual breathes the contaminated air. In addition, the process that occurs once the TB bacilli are in the lungs is largely determined by the individual's immune response. Seventy per cent of healthy TB contacts eradicate the bacilli and show no signs of infection (Health Protection Agency, 2005). Traditionally, tuberculosis has been associated with overcrowding, poor ventilation and limited sunlight because the bacilli are killed by ultraviolet radiation. In addition to inhalation, tuberculosis may also be transmitted by ingestion (particularly *M. bovis* in milk) or by accidental inoculation through the skin.

Activity

Make a list of things that may weaken a person's immune response and might make them more susceptible to infection.

- Pre-existing disease (diabetes; renal disease; anaemia)
- Chemotherapy or radiotherapy
- Immunological disorders (including HIV infection)
- Pregnancy
- Age (very young and very old)
- Nutritional status
- Stress

Box 16.1 Signs and symptoms

Pulmonary	General
Cough >3 weeks (dry or productive)	Tiredness, lethargy
Localised chest pain	Unexplained weight loss
Breathlessness	Fever, night sweats
Haemoptysis	Pain at affected site
Loss of appetite	

Diagnosis

Diagnosing tuberculosis is not always straightforward. A diagnosis is usually reached using a combination of clinical examination, investigations and tests. The signs and symptoms of tuberculosis are often indistinguishable from those associated with other diseases, and patients may present with non-specific complaints or vague respiratory illness that could have many other causes. In areas where tuberculosis is less common, this can lead to a delay in diagnosis and sometimes death.

The bacteriological investigation of tuberculosis is the only certain way of confirming a diagnosis. This is performed by microbiological detection of the tubercule bacillus, usually from a sputum specimen. The most frequent test is the examination of sputum smears after staining for acid-fast bacilli (AFB) (International Union Against Tuberculosis and Lung Disease, 2000). Sputum microscopy is critical in identifying infectious patients and therefore in the overall control of TB. Nurses have a key role in ensuring that high quality specimens are taken.

There is evidence that, of patients eventually found to be sputum smear positive, 80–90% are diagnosed on the first sputum specimen (Pratt *et al.*, 2005).

Where sputum is not readily available, fibre optic bronchoscopy may be used to obtain bronchial washings or biopsies. Specimens can also be obtained for histological examination. In children, gastric washings can be very effective, since children usually swallow their respiratory secretions. Renal tuberculosis is usually diagnosed from specimens of urine. Other specimens that can be used for bacteriological examination include pleural biopsies or fine-needle aspirates of tissue or exudates.

Box 16.2 Collection of sputum specimens

- Sputum (not saliva) is required – clear patient instruction is necessary
- The specimen should be collected *directly* into a sterile collection pot
- Clear labelling and packaging are important – 'biohazard' labels may be necessary
- Specimens should be transported to the laboratory with a minimum of delay
- Ideally, three specimens should be taken (on three consecutive days) to maximise the chance of detecting the bacilli
- Sputum produced during the first hour or two in the morning is ideal

> ## Point for thought
>
> Some of the most common problems with the simple process of collecting sputum specimens include:
>
> - Inadequate specimens (saliva, not sputum)
> - Improperly labelled or packaged specimens
> - Long delays in specimens reaching the laboratory
>
> Why do you think these things occur? How can they be avoided?

Following the initial AFB stain, specimens are cultured to identify the species of mycobacteria and perform drug susceptibility testing. Culture results may take several weeks to become available using traditional methods due to the slow-growing nature of mycobacteria. Rapid bacteriological methods are available and there have been new developments in molecular technology that now allow DNA 'fingerprinting'.

Radiological examination

The use of chest X-rays to support a diagnosis of tuberculosis continues to be widespread. Although this is a very sensitive tool for detecting pulmonary lesions, it is not always a very specific test since even large lung cavities may be suggestive of other pulmonary pathology, for example lung cancer. In addition, chest X-rays may be particularly difficult to interpret in HIV-infected people.

Tuberculin testing

Tuberculin skin tests are used to indicate whether an individual has an immunological reaction to mycobacterial antigens. Two types of tuberculin skin test may be used; the Heaf test or the Mantoux test. The differences are in the strength of tuberculin protein used and the method of administration. However, a positive tuberculin reaction is not considered to be diagnostic of TB, since reactivity can occur as a result of sensitisation by mycobacteria in the environment or by previous vaccination with Bacille Calmette-Guerin (BCG).

In addition, a negative response does not exclude active tuberculosis. People with severe immunosuppression due to advanced TB disease or HIV infection may have such weakened immune responses that they fail to react to the tuberculin protein.

Key point

The nursing care of people undergoing investigation for TB must be informed by knowledge of the complexity of reaching a diagnosis and an understanding of the anxiety that this may cause.

Tuberculosis is a notifiable disease. This means that a legal duty rests on the medical practitioners who attend people suspected of having tuberculosis to notify the names and addresses of these patients. Notifications in England and Wales are made to the Proper Officer of the local authority; local authorities are required to appoint such officers – usually the local Consultant in Health Protection. Notification is intended to support surveillance to detect potential outbreaks and it ensures that contact tracing occurs in order to find people at risk of exposure.

Isolation of known or suspected infectious patients

The isolation of patients in hospital must follow the locally agreed policy. Unless there is a clear clinical or socio-economic need, people with tuberculosis of any site of disease should not be admitted to hospital for diagnostic tests or care.

In general, anyone suspected as having pulmonary tuberculosis requiring hospital admission should be cared for in a single room vented to the air outside. People known to have respiratory tuberculosis must be separated from immuno-compromised patients, by admission either to a single room on a separate ward or to a negative pressure room on the same ward. Whilst ventilation dilutes airborne infectious particles, it does not contain them. Where it is essential to prevent contaminated air from an isolation room escaping through the door towards other patient areas, the air in the room must be at negative pressure and safely removed. Properly engineered negative pressure rooms have the air pressure continuously and automatically monitored, with windows that do not open and exhaust systems that remove the air safely to the outside.

Point for thought

Why do you think it is better to investigate people as outpatients and avoid hospital admission?

What advice would you give to someone with smear-positive pulmonary tuberculosis if they have been diagnosed with TB in the chest clinic and sent home to start treatment?

Summary of patient care in isolation rooms

- Patients must remain in the room with the door closed throughout the period of infectiousness and should not wander into communal areas.
- Universal infection control precautions apply (as they do to all patients), but inappropriate infection control measures must not be introduced; items contaminated with respiratory secretions *are not* associated with the transmission of *M. tuberculosis* and therefore disposable crockery and cutlery are not required. Patients may use general ward library services etc. No special precautions are required for rubbish, unless it is visibly contaminated with blood or body fluids
- The number of health care workers entering the room should be restricted to an appropriate minimum.
- While patients are infectious, visitors should be limited to those who have already been in contact with the patient prior to their diagnosis (including children). Visitors should be required to comply with infection control precautions.

Key point

The nursing care of people in isolation should pay particular attention to the social and psychological needs of patients.

Treatment

The medical treatment of tuberculosis aims to cure the disease and reduce the risk of transmission by rendering people non-infectious as quickly as possible.

Modern short-course anti-tuberculosis therapy is internationally standardised according to World Health Organization (WHO) guidelines.

In the UK, this means that two-phase therapy is used with a combination of four first-line drugs (Box 16.3).

Anti-tuberculosis drugs may be divided into two types: *bacteriostatic* agents, which can prevent the tubercle bacilli from duplication, and *bactericidal* agents, which kill the bacilli. It is important that TB treatment is standardised and that it is supervised by doctors and nurses with specialist knowledge of the disease in order to reduce the risk of drug-resistant organisms occurring.

Box 16.3 Standard Recommended Drug Regimen for Adults with Pulmonary Tuberculosis (British Thoracic Society, 1998)

Drug	Dose	Initial phase	Continuation phase
Isoniazid	300 mg daily	2 months	4 months
Rifampicin	Weight < 50 kg: 450 mg daily	2 months	4 months
	Weight > 50 kg: 600 mg daily		
Pyrazinamide	Weight < 50 kg: 1.5 g daily	2 months	Not applicable
	Weight > 50 kg: 2 g daily		
Ethambutol	15 mg/kg	2 months	Not applicable

NB: Combination preparations are usually prescribed to reduce the total number of tablets necessary; for example: Rifater® (rifampicin, isoniazid and pyrazinamide) or Rifinah® (rifampicin and isoniazid).

The nursing management of patients with tuberculosis

The role of the Specialist TB Nurse is divided into two main areas:

- caring for, monitoring and supporting patients on TB treatment
- coordinating the public health contact tracing activity

The patient

Because of the importance of taking anti-tuberculosis treatment correctly and consistently to achieve a cure and prevent drug resistance, adherence with therapy is paramount. Thus, nursing interventions to support and maintain treatment need to occur right from initial diagnosis. Early assessment will include the patient's psychological and social situation and serve to initiate a patient–nurse partnership.

The patient's knowledge, beliefs and understanding of their disease are key to developing strategies to support adherence. Information provided in appropriate ways enables people to take part in the decision-making process and to take individual responsibility for their contribution to clinical management. Despite the ability to cure tuberculosis, there remains a significant impact on clients' quality of life. Nurses involved in all stages of the care of people with TB should be mindful of how their management may influence ongoing concordance and treatment success.

The essential elements of an initial consultation with the specialist TB nurse are:

- Reassurance that tuberculosis is a treatable disease and can be cured
- Information about disease transmission, the level of infectivity and the requirements for isolation/restricting social contact
- Emphasising the importance of compliance with the treatment regime; information about the drugs and an explanation of how and why the medication needs to be taken
- Instruction on the potential adverse effects of treatment and emergency contact details for medical advise in the event of significant side-effects
- An explanation of the contact tracing process and the initiation of contact tracing (gathering important information about the health status of close contacts, establishing whether there are any particularly vulnerable contacts, such as babies or pregnant women, and finding out about workplace or school contacts)

Contact tracing

Contact tracing and the screening of contacts is usually organised by the specialist TB nurses. The purpose of contact tracing for tuberculosis is:

■ to discover people who may have become infected from the source case (but not yet developed active disease)
■ to discover any further cases of active tuberculosis disease
■ to discover anyone else who may have become infected from an unidentified source case

The aim of contact screening is to identify all the individuals who may be at increased risk from tuberculosis and investigate them appropriately. If latent infection is discovered, preventive treatment (chemoprophylaxis) may be given to prevent active cases occurring in the future.

In the UK, contact tracing protocols are guided by national recommendations (British Thoracic Society, 2000; National Institute for Health and Clinical Excellence, 2005)

Summary

Tuberculosis is one of the most common infectious diseases in the world. The global increase in TB cases is mainly occurring in developing countries but is also affecting the UK.

There should be a high index of suspicion for tuberculosis in patients who present with:

■ chronic cough
■ unexplained weight loss
■ fevers and/or night sweats
■ lethargy and tiredness
■ shortness of breath
■ chest pain
■ haemoptysis

Tuberculosis typically affects the lungs, but also commonly presents as extra-pulmonary tuberculosis (such as lymph gland, spinal or renal TB), especially in patients born outside the UK.

Globally, resistance to anti-tuberculous drugs is increasing. The best way to prevent resistance is to monitor and support patients to ensure that they complete the prescribed treatment meticulously.

All patients with tuberculosis should be Notified and should be clinically managed by a chest physician with specialist knowledge and training in TB. You should refer all patients with tuberculosis to the TB Nursing Service or Specialist TB Nurse.

References

Ait-Khaled, N. and Enarson, D. A. (2003) *Tuberculosis. A Manual for Medical Students*. World Health Organization, Geneva.

British Thoracic Society (1998) Chemotherapy and management of tuberculosis in the United Kingdom: recommendations 1998. *Thorax*, **53**, 536–48.

British Thoracic Society (2000) Control and prevention of tuberculosis in the United Kingdom: Code of Practice 2000. *Thorax*, **55**, 887–901.

Department of Health (2004) *Stopping Tuberculosis in England – An Action Plan from the Chief Medical Officer.* http://www.dh.gov/PolicyAndGuidance/HealthAndSocialCareTopics/Tuberculosis/fs/en/.

Health Protection Agency (2005) *Tuberculosis Factsheet for Schools.* http://www.hpa.org.uk/infections/topics_az/wfhfactsheets/WFHTB.htm.

Pratt JP. Grange MP. Williams VG. (2005) *Tuberculosis: A Foundation for Nursing & Healthcare Practice*. Hodder Arnold. London.

World Health Organization (2005). *World Health Organisation Global Tuberculosis Programme.* http://www.who.int/topics/tuberculosis/.

Web sites

International Union Against Tuberculosis and Lung Disease: http://www.iuatld.org/

TB Alert: http://www.tbalert.org.uk/

UK Department of Health Action Plan: http://www.dh.gov.uk/PolicyAndGuidance/HealthAndSocialCareTopics/Tuberculosis/

National Institute of Health and Clinical Excellence Tuberculosis Clinical Guidelines – second consultation: http://www.nice.org.uk/page.aspx?o=271279.

Index